Agility in Health Care

Steven L. Goldman
Carol B. Graham
Editors

Foreword by Jeff Goldsmith

Agility in Health Care

Strategies for Mastering Turbulent Markets

Sponsored by Agility Forum

Jossey-Bass Publishers
San Francisco

Jossey-Bass books and products are available through most bookstores. To contact Jossey-Bass directly, call (888) 378-2537, fax to (800) 605-2665, or visit our website at www.josseybass.com.

Substantial discounts on bulk quantities of Jossey-Bass books are available to corporations, professional associations, and other organizations. For details and discount information, contact the special sales department at Jossey-Bass.

For sales outside the United States, please contact your local Simon & Schuster International Office.

Manufactured in the United States of America using Lyons Falls D'Anthology paper, which is a special blend of non-tree fibers and totally chlorine-free wood pulp.

Library of Congress Cataloging-in-Publication Data

Agility in health care : strategies for mastering turbulent markets / edited by Steven L. Goldman and Carol B. Graham. — 1st ed.
p. cm. — (The Jossey-Bass health series)
Includes bibliographical references (p.) and index.
ISBN 0-7879-4211-1 (cloth)
1. Health maintenance organizations—Miscellanea. 2. Competition. 3. Organizational change. 4. Customer services. I. Goldman, Steven L., 1941– II. Graham, Carol B., 1947– III. Series.
RA413 .A34 1999
362.1'04258—ddc21 98-40111

HB Printing 10 9 8 7 6 5 4 3 2 1 FIRST EDITION

Contents

Foreword

It has been a difficult decade for those who sought easy transference of management wisdom and models from the corporate world into the American health care system. Not that health care managers are not ready and eager to master a new private language or sign up for the latest fad. Futurist Ian Morrison has dubbed the seemingly inexhaustible well of new management jargon and concepts "lemmingware." Yet the track record for corporate models transplanted into the health care world has been grim. Portfolio management, diversification, multidivisional corporate structures, matrix management: the list seems endless. Why have the results been so disappointing?

Part of the problem is the sheer complexity of health care as a business, and of the health care transaction itself. Nowhere else in the American economy is there more variability or uncertainty at the point of service than in the health care transaction. Nor will one find a comparable density of expert professionals colliding at the point of service. No less a management authority than Peter Drucker has asserted that the large urban hospital is probably the single most complex human institution. Organizational complexity and the anarchic influence of professional values and cultures have conspired to render management models derived from manufacturing or other service industries inadequate.

So why should agility fare any differently? Simply because health care enterprises are in serious danger of losing touch with their customers. As the merger movement has accelerated through the world of health plans, hospitals, physician groups, and health product suppliers, the distance between those who run health care enterprises and the ultimate beneficiary of their efforts, the American consumer, has grown insupportably large.

Health care organizations have been busily rendering themselves less agile, patterning their strategies on organizational templates that no longer work in the manufacturing and retail sectors where they originated. As they have become less responsive, their cost and management structures have become a major impediment to profitable operation. Boards and management that expected economies of scale and coordination from a larger asset base have experienced crippling diseconomies, as well as increasing political exposure. Few health care managers realize that the management template they are copying is literally bankrupt. It no longer works in the economic sectors that invented it, forcing manufacturing firms to rethink fundamentally and reinvent an operating logic for the new economy.

Reconnecting with the "end user" is an urgent priority for all health care enterprises, an urgency that has grown into a marketing imperative as health plans offer broader choice of providers to their subscribers. The reassertion of consumer choice as a fundamental principle in health care organization comes at a time when both health plans and delivery organizations seem to be striving to narrow or eliminate choice through their corporate strategies. Consumers are sending the health system a fundamentally different message than are the corporate strategists who advise health system leadership, and those organizations that truly listen to the customer rather than the management gurus will be the ones that prosper in the increasingly retail market for health services.

Americans resent the emerging corporate face of medicine, and have expressed their wrath not only in an angry backlash against managed care but against health care corporations generally. With increasing urgency, American consumers have insisted on being architects of their own health care experience. They do not want anyone—employer, health plan, health system, or government—telling them who they will see to resolve their complex problems. What agility demands of any organization, health care or otherwise, is active listening to the customer and those who collaborate in meeting the customer's needs. Agility also demands an immediate, custom-tailored solution to those needs.

Health care enterprises have begun to adopt a new, more flexible model—a virtual organization model that is based not on ownership, but on collaboration among enterprises with complementary skill sets and capabilities. As the chapters in this book establish, this new collaborative model of value creation is not easy to master, particularly in a field such as health services where collaboration has been so little accepted. Virtual organization strategies are no panacea. They are relationship dependent and require a degree of internal discipline and cohesion that will test the partners in any effective collaboration.

But the discipline that agility and the virtual organization model require is vitally needed in health enterprises. "Being virtual" requires a degree of organizational realism and self-knowledge that has not been required before—a capacity to identify core competencies and the organizational capacity to discontinue strategies, programs, or services that do not offer unique value to the consumer of health services. Successfully executed, however, agility helps simplify an organization and help it focus its physical and human capital on the areas where it can produce the greatest return and the solutions of greatest value to the customer. For health care enterprises, agility is an idea whose time has come.

Jeff Goldsmith
Health Futures, Inc.
Charlottesville, West Virginia

Preface

In May 1996, I delivered a speech on the new realities of industrial agility-based competition at a conference for health care leaders organized by Andersen Consulting. I don't know who was more surprised: me, when Andersen partner Dave Blume first asked me to join with noted health care consultant Jeff Goldsmith in leading off the conference, or the audience, who found themselves listening to a presentation on a profit-based model of commerce that was derived from manufacturing.

During the preceding four years, I had given lectures, seminars, and workshops on agility to over one hundred corporate audiences across industry sectors, but to the best of my knowledge, this was the first invitation anyone had received to address health care executives on the subject. Fortunately, once the connection was made, the relevance of agility to the concerns of health care professionals was obvious.

I challenged the Andersen audience to translate to their own areas of expertise the agility model that was then so successfully transforming U.S. industry: selling solutions rather than discrete products and services; developing collaborative relationships with customers, suppliers, partners, and even competitors; creating an adaptive organizational structure and an entrepreneurial workforce; and leveraging competencies, information, and knowledge to create competitive advantages. Over the next two days, these health care leaders—few, if any, of whom had heard of agility before—did just that. Speakers and panelists repeatedly referred to the similarity between the forces that were driving change in manufacturing and those driving change in the U.S. health care system. More to the point, people were excited by the prospect of applying to health care the specific responses of industry to those drivers. Some highly respected health care experts, among them Jeff Goldsmith and Henry Ford Health Systems corporate vice president Vinod Sahney, identified agility as the new strategic framework within which health care organizations needed to position themselves.

Almost exactly a year later, I delivered a keynote address at the Healthier Communities Summit organized by the Health Care Forum, whose director, Kathryn Johnson, had attended the Andersen conference a year earlier. In that 1997 address, I was able to relate agility to a growing body of experience that my Agility Forum colleague Carol Graham and I were acquiring by applying agility concepts to a broad range of health care organizations: payers, providers, educators, and suppliers. The Healthier Communities Summit audience was ten times the size of the Andersen conference audience—two thousand compared to two hundred—but the agility model no longer came as a surprise to them.

In the intervening year, events in the health care world—especially the continuing growth of for-profit hospital networks and managed care enterprises, and increasingly painful competition and cost pressure that is affecting everyone, from drug and equipment manufacturers to teaching hospitals—had intensified the need for a strategic approach to "reengineering" health care. The Health Care Forum audience was not willing to settle for being challenged by a new idea. They wanted to hear how agility could be *applied* to health care enterprises, how the model developed by the Agility Forum could help them in their organizations to function better in a suddenly chaotic, openly profit-driven, and relentlessly cost-sensitive health care environment.

What in 1991 my colleagues and I had named "agility" was increasingly being recognized as the key to the astonishing turnaround in the global competitiveness of U.S. industry. The increasingly obvious new health care reality was that health care was, economically, just another industry. For the first time since the reforms instigated by the World War I–era Flexner report, every element of the U.S. health care system, especially the delivery of care, was fully exposed to prevailing market forces.

The unique intimacy of the doctor-patient relationship, the privileged position of the physician as the unchallengeable arbiter of care decisions, and the right of the patients to make treatment choices based on what they deem to be in their best interest are all rapidly fading memories. In the health care world, as in the corporate world, economic rationality rules. Today every activity within the health care system must be justified in economic terms, and every health care organization is struggling to meet that challenge. The difficulty of doing so is complicated by marketplace changes that have redefined the economic rationality to which health care organizations must adapt.

Under unprecedented pressure from foreign competitors and changing marketplace values, American companies in the mid–1980s began a lengthy process of reinventing themselves. Painfully, they discovered what the new marketplace realities were as they created responses to them. Inevitably, the process was inefficient. Management blamed labor, and labor blamed management. Industrial leaders, union officials, and politicians blamed unfair foreign competition and demanded government action to "level the playing field." Experts held out foreign competitors as models to be emulated, praising the social institutions and cultural values to which the economic miracles of these competitors were attributed. Critics assailed the values of the marketplace. Consultants offered "success pills" that executives raced one another to buy and install first: just-in-time operations, continuous improvement, quality circles, matrix organizations, teaming, empowerment, visionary leadership, Total Quality Management, learning organizations, and reengineering.

By the early 1990s, a new model for global commerce began to emerge from these piecemeal efforts of hundreds of companies, each seeking to gain or reclaim competitive advantage in their changing markets. The model was given the name *agility* and emerged first in manufacturing. GE, Chrysler, IBM, Motorola, Xerox, Hewlett-Packard, Texas Instruments, Caterpillar, Boeing, Compaq, Dell, and Gateway, among many others, began restoring the competitiveness, and the profitability, of U.S. industry after a decade of decline.

This reversal happened by organizing the production of goods and services around the fact that the center of marketplace value had shifted from manufacturing to information and services. Acknowledging this fact and responding to it required a fundamental change in managerial values and strategic thinking. In markets that valued information and services highly, it was the organization of resources, and not the resources themselves, that determined competitive success. The organizational structures suited to stable, mass markets that valued products were not suited to rapidly changing niche markets that valued information and services. Agility opened up a new space for rethinking how to organize which resources to compete successfully in the most profitable new growth markets.

The ideas underlying agility were first described in a 1991 report I had coauthored with Kenneth Preiss that was published by the Iacocca Institute at Lehigh University. Over the next two and a half years, an astonishing thirty thousand copies of that report were sold. In 1994, Iacocca Institute director Roger Nagel, Kenneth Preiss, and I wrote *Agile Competitors and Virtual Organizations: Strategies for Enriching the Customer*, which contained over one hundred illustrations of applications of agility concepts in U.S. companies. That book was one of four finalists for best American management book of 1995 and has been translated into ten languages, including Japanese, in which it was a business best-seller. In 1996, with the same colleagues, I coauthored *Cooperate to Compete: Building Agile Business Relationships*. This book focuses on implementing agility in extended enterprises—networks of collaborating companies—that we called "interprises." In their own ways, using their own names to describe it—*agile*, *nimble*, *high velocity*—companies around the world have been fundamentally transforming how they produce goods and services and how they market, distribute, and price them.

It is hardly surprising that people and organizations adapted to a health care system that was to a significant degree sheltered from the commercial marketplace are struggling mightily today. They have to assimilate a wholly commercial mind-set at a time when commercial values are themselves in a state of flux. But people and organizations coming into health care from the commercial sector are struggling too. They want to apply to health care companies the competitiveness lessons that industry has learned, and they are finding success elusive. They want to create health care companies that operate in the new way that commercial enterprises do, but health care companies are largely unaware of this new mode of operation.

One obstacle for both groups is that people in the health care sector do not relate the changes they are experiencing to the changes that have taken place in the industrial sector. They are nevertheless being subjected to the same drivers of change to which first manufacturing and then services have been subjected over the past fifteen years. And they are responding as industry initially did. Each organization is attempting piecemeal implementations of the same "success pill" tactics that commercial enterprises adopted.

This book is a response to that situation. Our goal in writing it is to create a shared understanding of agility among health care professionals and businesspeople who together are trying to establish a high-quality health care system based on prevailing commercial values. In the chapters that follow, we address four subjects:

1. What an agile organization is
2. Why health care professionals are excited by the prospect of implementing agility
3. How readers can assess the value of agility to their organization
4. How organizations can use agility to convert marketplace threats into growth opportunities

Chapter One describes the organizational capabilities that define an agile enterprise, with illustrations of how agility is being implemented in industry. Health care organizations, struggling to adapt to unfamiliar market forces and values, will benefit in two ways from paying careful attention to these non–health care illustrations. First, they validate agility as an organizational model. Second, they are a seedbed of innovative ideas, showing the many ways that companies across the economy are successfully reinventing themselves as agile enterprises.

In Chapters Two through Eight, health care professionals describe initiatives within and among health care organizations that reveal the movement of the health care system toward agility:

- Substituting alliances for traditional own-it-all integration
- Offering individualized customer solutions in place of discrete services
- Creating networks of win-win inter-enterprise relationships in place of opportunistic hierarchies
- Exploiting the power of information technologies to create value
- Sharing knowledge to competitive advantage
- Incorporating new marketplace realities into the training of the next generation of physicians

These initiatives confirm that the forces to which health care organizations are responding are the same ones that have been driving industry to embrace agility. It follows that organizational change in the health care system can be accomplished more effectively, and less painfully, by building on the experience of industry.

Chapter Nine presents a simple tool set that readers can use to outline a migration strategy to agility for themselves and their organizations.

Those within the health care system and those attempting to become part of it are seeking to bring to the health care marketplace a new solution to the problem of satisfying a diverse, demanding, and rapidly changing spectrum of stakeholder interests. Agility has emerged as a basis for such a solution in industry, which has already climbed a painful learning curve, similar to the one that health care organizations are climbing now. Corporations, exposed to relentless competitive pressures and increasingly demanding stakeholder expectations, have found in agility a means of improving their competitiveness and meeting those expectations. Health care organizations cannot afford to dismiss what they have found on the grounds that health care is "different." It *was* different, once; now it is distinctive as a *service* but with similarities as a *business* that compel learning from the experiences of those who have paid the high price of learning for themselves.

August 1998
Bethlehem, Pennsylvania Steven L. Goldman

Acknowledgments

We express our appreciation to the chapter authors for their willingness to assimilate the agility paradigm to their evolving expertise, as well as for accepting the unrealistic deadlines we asked them to meet; and to our Jossey-Bass editor, Andrew Pasternack, whose support, assistance, and good judgment moved this book from idea to reality. We owe special thanks to Carolyn Uno of Tigris Productions; to Ralph Sorrell, former CEO of Lake Hospital System in Painesville, Ohio, who gave us our first opportunity to apply the Agility Forum's model and tools to a health care organization, one that Ralph had built into a formidable competitor; and to Agility Forum CEO Rusty Patterson for allowing us to use forum-generated materials in preparing this book. Interested readers can consult the forum's web site: www.agilityforum.org.

Steven L. Goldman
Carol B. Graham

The Editors

Steven L. Goldman is Andrew W. Mellon Distinguished Professor in the Humanities at Lehigh University in Bethlehem, Pennsylvania. He is coauthor of the 1991 report that introduced the term *agile competition* and first presented a detailed vision of post–mass production commerce. Goldman is one of the founders of the Agility Forum, a nonprofit corporation established jointly by U.S. industry and government to accelerate the transition to agility-based commerce. He served for two years as the forum's chief operating officer and chief technical officer, returning in 1997 to his academic position and creating Agility Consulting Services as a means of developing his ideas about effective organizational transformation in an agile competitive environment. He lectures widely and conducts customized interactive seminars and workshops, helping companies discover how to leverage agility selectively to their specific advantage. He can be reached at sgoldman@fast.net.

Carol B. Graham is a senior consultant with the Agility Forum, working closely with Steve Goldman in the development, application, and implementation of the agility model and tools in the health care industry. She has worked with community-based hospitals, academic medical centers, colleges and universities, payer organizations, and government agencies. She specializes in the development and cultivation of agile relationships between and among health care organizations and organizations in other industries to implement collaborative programs that identify mutually beneficial solutions. She also works with Steve Goldman to develop and conduct workshops and assessments designed to help health care organizations improve customer service, develop value-added customized products, and achieve new levels of leadership excellence. She can be reached at cgraham@agilityforum.net.

The Contributors

Michael H. Annison is president of the Westrend Group in Denver, a consultancy that monitors social, economic, and political change in the United States, and author of *Managing the Whirlwind: Patterns and Opportunities in a Changing World.* Prior to forming the Westrend Group, he was vice president of the Naisbitt Group, whose research was the basis for the book *Megatrends*. His experience in the field of health care has included work with the Estes Park Institute, the board of the American Hospital Association, national and state long-term care groups, and more than one hundred hospitals and health care systems.

Michael W. Barton is founder, chairman, president, and chief executive officer of PriCare, Inc., a physician practice management company headquartered in Brentwood, Tennessee. PriCare is the third company Barton has founded. In 1981, he cofounded Hospital Management Professionals, which became the second largest manager of not-for-profit hospitals in the United States. In 1991, he cofounded Health Horizons, an outpatient surgery center company of which he currently serves as chairman of the board.

Leanne Kaiser Carlson is an associate with Kaiser & Associates and a member of the International Health Futures Network, an alliance of leading futurists and health care organizations. She is cofounder of the Kaiser Technology Group, which focuses on Internet and intranet development for health care organizations. She writes and speaks extensively on the future of health care, demand management, technology, and the design of healthy communities. In addition to her consulting work, Kaiser is a faculty member of the Estes Park Institute and the Health Care Forum's Healthier Communities Fellowship.

James R. Cramer is vice president and chief information officer at Scottsdale Health Care in Scottsdale, Arizona. Before joining Scottsdale Health Care, he was a partner with Ernst & Young in Phoenix. He is a member of the Health Care Information and Management Systems Society and has served as president of the Technology and Information Management Education Society and of the Arizona Health Information Network.

Roderick Gilkey is executive director of the Center for Health Care Leadership at Emory University, where he holds joint appointments in the School of Medicine and the Goizueta School of Business. He conducts research on leadership, change management, and international negotiation, and is coauthor of *Joining Forces: Successfully Managing Mergers and Acquisitions*. Gilkey has provided consulting and executive education services to a broad array of global and Fortune 500 companies.

Scott Hendrickson is an information architect with Kaiser Technology Group. His experience includes modeling of complex dynamical systems, simulation and visualization software design and implementation, and Internet and intranet communication systems design and implementation. He has been involved in electronic commerce strategic planning, clinical guideline automation, and a number of object-oriented analysis and design projects. He is working on a system for personalized health care information delivery.

Martyn W. C. Howgill is the chief marketing officer at the University of Texas M. D. Anderson Cancer Center. He is a recognized expert in change management, reengineering, quality and work redesign, marketing, strategic planning, internal and external communications execution, and human resource issues. He has worked with health care organizations and institutions of higher education in the United States, Canada, and Great Britain.

Gary R. Lieberman is associate director of the Center for Health Care Leadership. He has provided consulting and education services on health care–related topics to organizations such as Merck, IBM, Vitalink, Emory Health Care, and the Medical College of Georgia. He currently teaches at the School of Medicine and the Goizueta School of Business at Emory University.

Wendy H. Lyons is vice president of health system integration for Scottsdale Health Care in Scottsdale, Arizona, where she focuses on community outreach for health care services, population health management, and continuous quality improvement activities. She has authored articles and given presentations on information technology in health care communications and nursing management structures. She works extensively with a number of community organizations in greater Scottsdale to promote education on healthy lifestyles.

David B. Nash is founding director of the Office of Health Policy and Clinical Outcomes at Thomas Jefferson University, associate dean for health policy and associate professor of medicine at Jefferson Medical College in Philadelphia, and associate director of the Partnerships for Quality Education program. His work in outcomes management, medical staff development, and quality-of-care improvement has been widely published in more than forty journals and ten books, including *The Physician's Guide to Managed Care* and *A Systems Approach to Disease Management*.

Martin N. Raber is professor of medicine and vice president for managed care and outreach programs at the University of Texas M. D. Anderson Cancer Center in Houston. He also serves as chairman of the board of directors of the M. D. Anderson Physicians Network. Raber is working on the development of new health care delivery systems for cancer patients, managed care contracting strategies for specialty institutions, and the assessment of quality and outcomes in the management of cancer.

Morton D. Sosland has written numerous articles on business and health care. He received his bachelor's degree in economics from Harvard University and his M.B.A. in marketing from the Wharton School. He holds a master's degree in international studies from the University of Pennsylvania and is currently a medical student at Jefferson Medical College.

1

Agility for Health Care

Who Ordered That?

Steven L. Goldman

What is an agile organization, and why are so many health care leaders interested in agility?

An organization is agile if, by leveraging knowledge and cooperation, it is able to thrive in rapidly changing, intensely competitive markets that place a high value on information-and service-based products, called *solutions*, tailored to the needs of individual customers. There is no universal formula for becoming agile. Nor is there a technology to buy or a technique to master; no one will find seven or twelve steps to guaranteed success.

"Agile" is shorthand for a complex, context-sensitive organizational capability. It is the capability to coordinate quickly and efficiently all of the physically and organizationally distributed resources required to create, produce, deliver, and support a constantly changing mix of goods and services for fickle markets.

To be agile is to be prepared, in advance of customers' expressed needs, to provide them with goods and services whose value in part lies in having them available on demand, when the demand arises. To do this routinely requires totally different capabilities from those that made for corporate success in the past. Agility requires an unprecedented degree of organizational and operational flexibility. It requires a continuing engagement with the social and economic forces affecting the behavior and the changing requirements of individual customers. It requires accepting new levels of risk: sharing sensitive information with suppliers, partners, and customers; anticipating marketplace change and customer values; operating as close to real time as possible, with minimal buffers of inventory, production capacity, and personnel. Above all, to be agile is to be able to integrate selectively people and processes, knowledge and skills, regardless of their organizational location, within a company or in other companies: suppliers, partners, or even customers themselves.

Think for a moment about the implications of this complex of capabilities for the health care system. Before exploring in greater detail the attributes of an agile organization, does agility sound like something that a health care organization today—a provider organization, a payer organization, vendors, researchers, a medical school—might find valuable? On the face of it, the quality and the cost-effectiveness of health care delivery, and thus its profitability, could only be improved if health care enterprises were organized around the objective of customer-driven win-win relationships in place of the currently popular shareholder-driven winner-take-all strategies. Consider the following handful of initiatives that health care organizations are pursuing.

Tenet Health Care, with 131 acute care hospitals, has an annual supply budget of $1.2 billion. It has created a decentralized network of vested panels of doctors and nurses at its hospitals who have the authority to identify the suppliers they wish to use for many high clinical preference supplies. Tenet has motivated responsibility and accountability by pushing decisions down to the appropriate operational level, and it has concurrently improved the efficiency and reduced the cost of the operational processes involved.

Emory University, Ohio State, Northwestern, and the University of Pennsylvania have formed the virtual Academy for Health Care Quality that draws on resources distributed across those institutions to offer national continuing education and training programs for health care professionals. Emory and its partners have broken through organizational boundaries that traditionally fenced off expertise, to integrate a focused set of complementary resources into a solution in whose benefits all share.

Aetna/U.S. Healthcare is pooling data from 14 million members who had been contained in five different and incompatible software systems covering thirteen regional markets into a single data warehouse. This data pooling will allow Aetna to link claims information to data on providers, premiums, finances, and employers. At the same time, it creates an evolving medical database that is a valuable product in its own right to managed care organizations and traditional indemnity plans. In just one attempt at exploring how to use this information effectively, Aetna has given $6 million in research grants to thirteen academic institutions to study the best treatment strategies for medically underserved populations. Aetna is leveraging information to create new knowledge products.

Shared Medical Systems and Crozer-Keystone Hospital System, headquartered in Upland, Pennsylvania, have developed the Physicians Office of the Future in whose design, unusual by past practices, physicians played a central role. In addition to the comprehensive integration of all of the business and medical information needs of over three hundred physicians in over two hundred offices in the southwestern Pennsylvania–northern Delaware region, the physicians are linked to a comprehensive central hospital systems database covering 550,000 patients. Software allows data analysis relating to efficiency of care and care profiles. The system is being extended to include productivity and case mix analyses. Crozier-Keystone is creating an integrated information infrastructure that enables everyone in the system to use information and knowledge to create customer-specific solutions.

Florida-based FHP International has spun off its network of owned clinics in order to attract business from other health plans. Similarly, Kaiser Permanente, whose strategic plan in the mid–1980s called for spending billions to build or update facilities, is contracting with other hospital systems to manage or assume ownership of Kaiser facilities and scaling back, or even terminating, operations at others. FHP and Kaiser are following the shift in marketplace value to focused competencies, facilitating the most effective delivery of health care services rather than owning the facilities that deliver them.

From a very narrow perspective, some health care providers can claim to have been agile for a long time. A hospital emergency room, after all, sounds very much like an agile organization. Patients arrive unpredictably with specific problems that typically bear no relationship to the problems of the immediately preceding or following patients. A small staff of highly trained people work cooperatively, self-configuring the range of skills and knowledge appropriate for responding to each patient's needs. They reach out, as those needs require, to engage the wider pool of expertise available within the emergency room, in the hospital, on call, in other hospitals, and even worldwide, through global medical databases and access to superstar specialists and researchers.

The agility of the emergency room is, however, a special case. It is the product of a mission rather than of market forces. But imagine a hospital, a rehabilitation facility, a managed care enterprise, a medical device or pharmaceuticals manufacturer, or a national health care system whose routine operations were as dynamic, as collaborative, and as customer centered as the emergency room's. This may sound implausible given today's health care realities. And yet U.S. industry has implemented just such a new global system of market-pulled production in less than ten years. The health care industry *can* do the same. Will it?

The Problem to Which Agility Is the Solution

U.S. industry adopted the organizational capabilities called agility not because they seemed to be a good idea but as a compelling solution to two problems that confronted them with increasing urgency in the course of the 1980s: the immediate problem, which was forcing fundamental change in the way that commercial enterprises were operated, and the *real* problem, of forcing change in the way that they were organized and managed.

The immediate problem was that the target of commercial competition had shifted. Until the 1980s, the greatest profit target was standardized mass market products and services that had long market lifetimes, were produced to forecast, and had a sales price determined by production costs plus a markup limited by competitors' marketing practices.

Beginning in the 1980s, and at an accelerating rate, the target became niche market solutions that are individualized, have a short market life, are produced to order in a wide range of constantly changing variations, and have a value that is determined by continuing relationships with customers. This is at least as profound a shift in the foundations of business as the one that occurred after the creation of the modern corporation at the end of the nineteenth century. Then, hundreds of thousands of small businesses serving local markets suddenly found themselves in competition with remote, giant national businesses able to offer their local customers much greater variety and at much lower prices. These new corporate competitors were exploiting economies of scope and scale and concentrations of resources that were unavailable to local businesses. Today the real problem threatening businesses of all sizes comes from two directions, both emanating from the marketplace rather than from the executive suite: the pace of change and the center of value.

The pace of change in mainstream commercial competition, the most profitable markets for goods and services, has outstripped the functionality of inherited management tools. The management model, the organizational structure, and the business processes that served corporations so well for so long no longer work well. They are not flexible enough, not responsive enough, not knowledge centered enough to fulfill the expectations of today's customers for constant streams of new models of existing products and for new kinds of products.

In effect, the marketplace has redefined what a product is. The center of marketplace value has shifted decisively from goods to information and services, even within manufacturing. The traditional distinction between goods and services has been blurred by the strategy of selling goods *as* services, along with the strategy of selling goods in order to sell services. At the same time, there has been an enormous expansion in the number of companies whose only product is information.

For many years now, CEO Jack Welch has impressed on GE personnel that GE is not a manufacturing company—the locomotives, jet engines, and steam turbines they make notwithstanding. GE is a service company that manufactures things as a service to its customers. Selling a thing is a once-and-done-with deal. Selling a service is the beginning of a potentially long-term selling relationship. Welch is not talking here about what we normally mean by "servicing" a product, that is, repairing it if and when it breaks.

The services that Welch and his corporate peers at IBM, Hewlett-Packard, Johnson Controls, Honeywell, Boeing, and hundreds of other companies that make up the core of what are traditionally thought of as U.S. manufacturing want to sell are knowledge-based services that can create continuing, large, high-margin-income streams.

Steelcase Furniture advertises, "We manufacture desks, chairs, file cabinets and credenzas. Of course that's not what we sell." What Steelcase sells is expertise in creating effective office environments. Digital Equipment Corporation's (DEC) banking equipment division's most profitable sales are for branch bank design services, including the installation of automatic teller machines (ATMs) and printing equipment they buy from DEC and training of bank staff in its use and maintenance. Compaq Computer's surprising January 1998 bid to purchase DEC was motivated in part by the need for the knowledge DEC engineers have in designing minicomputers and in part by DEC's very successful computer services business, which brings in $6 billion a year.

Installing, maintaining, and upgrading computer hardware, software, and networks for corporate clients is a never-ending business. That is why IBM, Hewlett-Packard, and Unisys, along with DEC, so aggressively promote themselves as information services companies, not just computer manufacturers. Like Steelcase, they *manufacture* physical products, but that is not what they *sell*. What they sell are solutions to each customer's individual information processing needs. And they are quite willing to accommodate a customer's demand that the equipment component of that solution come from a rival manufacturer—regrettable, perhaps, when customers insist, but the services component of such integrated solutions usually amounts to 75 to 80 percent of the value of the contract. Clearly knowledge-based services wag the manufactured product tail.

Johnson Controls began as a thermostat manufacturer, and until recently its automotive division manufactured seats to precise specifications from GM, Ford, and Chrysler engineers. Today Johnson Controls has a multibillion dollar commercial building systems services division, and its more than six hundred automotive division engineers codesign auto and truck interiors with their Big Three engineer peers. They still manufacture seats, but now they ship them on a three-hour order cycle, delivering the seats directly to the point on the assembly line at which they are installed into the individual vehicle for which they have been ordered. The savings in inventory and assembly costs are what convert manufacturing into a service in this supplier-manufacturer relationship.

The common denominator behind the sudden discovery that services are where the profit and growth are is the growing market value of knowledge and information. This is one strong link between health care and industrial organizations today. It is further support for paying attention to how industrial companies are reorganizing so that they can become knowledge- and information-driven enterprises. It is not only that knowledge and information are increasingly salable products in their own right and increasingly necessary to create the solutions that are the heart of marketplace competitiveness. Only a knowledge- and information-driven enterprise can be agile, with the speediness of response to market opportunities, the flexibility, the innovativeness, and the adaptability to thrive in today's marketplace.

Management Challenges of Agility

A number of distinctive management challenges confront organizations striving to be agile:

- Knowing the business they are really in
- Perpetual solution creation
- Constant self-interrogation
- Managing knowledge
- Motivating the entire workforce

Knowing the Business They Are Really In

Management must challenge personnel to ask the questions, "What business are we *really* in?" "What are our customers *really* buying from us?" "What business *ought* we to be in, knowing what our customers value?" And management must be prepared to redefine the company, if necessary, depending on the answers to these questions, which, in rapidly changing markets, must be raised over and over again. The constant anchoring of this posture of continual preparedness for change is the goal of identifying and exploiting the highest market value competency that the company possesses.

These questions do not have obvious answers. Nor can businesses simply ask customers to answer them, though the answers always come ultimately from an understanding of customers. Often customers are not explicitly aware of what is most valuable to them in the combination of goods and services they buy. That is why under the agility paradigm, companies must be proactive in learning what customers do value and would value if it were offered to them. Remember that no one asked for music CDs, ATMs, or self-service gas stations.

The need to challenge the essential basis of a successful business rarely arose during most of the twentieth century. The pace of marketplace change was so leisurely, compared to today, that projecting the present form of the business into the future was the reasonable thing to do. That is no longer the case. The only defense against being threatened by change is to embrace its inevitability and be ready to adapt to it selectively. Responding successfully to this challenge holds such great potential for growth that it is worth looking at a number of illustrations from industry that may stimulate thinking about reinventing health care organizations.

What business is a health care organization really in? Consider the case of an insurer. Should it own clinics, hospitals, and practices? FHP and Kaiser Permanente, among others, are reexamining the logic of decisions that were right yesterday in answering yes, but that may not be right for tomorrow.

In 1982, ambulatory surgery accounted for less than 20 percent of all surgical procedures. By 1987, this had grown to 44 percent. In 1997, over 80 percent of surgical procedures were either outpatient or required fewer than two days of hospitalization. In the nation's largest managed care plan, Kaiser Permanente, an enrollee on average stays in a hospital once every sixteen years. Wills Eye Hospital in Philadelphia experienced this inpatient-to-outpatient shift in the form of growth in ambulatory eye surgery. It responded to the progressive underutilization of its large center city hospital facility by opening twelve satellite outpatient centers in the greater Philadelphia area. In its large center city hospital, Wills has leased the eighth floor to a geriatric psychiatric program and developed, jointly with nearby Jefferson and Pennsylvania hospitals, a virtual neurosurgical service that uses Wills staff and facilities and is now, even without the participation of Pennsylvania Hospital, which has joined the University of Pennsylvania Hospital System, the largest neurosurgical service on the East Coast.

These developments compel asking the question, "What business is a hospital *really* in today?" Should health professional staff be employees or contractors? Should the hospital own medical practices and compete with independent doctors? Does a hospital deliver care, or does it provide the infrastructure to facilitate the delivery of care? What business is a medical school in, or a diagnostic center, or a medical research institute?

The answers to these questions are no longer as obvious as they may have seemed as recently as ten years ago. What customers value most has changed, from products and services to individualized solutions. Inevitably the value that individual organizations can most cost-effectively contribute to the creation of those solutions has changed too. As a result, it is not even obvious what business pharmaceutical companies, medical device manufacturers, or health care–focused information services companies are in anymore. That is, it is not obvious how they should be harnessing their core competencies to the production of the combination of goods and services that niche markets value most highly. Examples of commercial enterprises that have successfully reinvented themselves challenge health care organizations to match their boldness.

What business is an electric utility in? This was a silly question until the mid–1990s, when this industry, which had been sheltered from prevailing market forces, was suddenly exposed to them. From Edison's creation of the industry in 1882 on, electric utilities had been integrated providers of electricity. They built power plants to generate electricity; bought rights-of-way over which to string power lines to transmit the electricity to their markets; distributed the electricity right into each customer's home, office, or business; and engaged in research, marketing, sales, and service activities.

Until the oil price shocks of the mid–1970s, utility executives automatically assumed that their historic 7 percent annual demand growth would continue indefinitely. Even as this growth rate collapsed under consumer and corporate conservation efforts, they committed to aggressive power plant construction programs intended to double their capacity to meet the anticipated higher demand. For the next twenty years, turbulent years for the utilities, they were insulated by their status as regulated public monopolies from market forces that were driving manufacturing toward agility. In the mid–1990s, however, came deregulation. Suddenly, the previously silly question, "What business *are* we in?" became the one on whose answer the future of the company depended. The answers have been revealing.

Some utilities have sold off their power plants and transmission lines and redefined themselves as electric distribution and service companies. Analogously, some integrated health care insurers, such as Kaiser Permanente, are divesting themselves of their hospitals or hiring companies to manage those hospitals for them. Some utilities redefined themselves as electricity generators only, buying power plants across the country and abandoning transmission lines and end-user marketing, sales, and service functions. Some have become marketing companies, buying electricity on the now-open market and contracting with transmission companies to deliver it to distributors with whom they have contracted to provide so much power at a fixed price. Of those that have chosen to be in the transmission business, some have begun asking if it is only electricity that they are positioned to transmit. Their distribution network, after all, reaches into virtually every building in the nation. Might the electricity transmission and distribution network be adaptable to providing telecommunications services, for example?

In fact, this very question had already been answered by a cousin utility several years earlier. Williams Companies is one of the nation's leading natural gas transporters. As telecommunications boomed in the late 1980s following the breakup of AT&T and the exponential growth in the volume of business data services, Williams's management asked what business they were really in. Of course, the company was a gas transporter, and a very profitable one, but was it only a *gas* transporter? Once the question was asked, the answer was obvious: no. By running fiber-optic cable through the national gas pipeline network that it already owned, Williams almost overnight became a leading long-distance business data transmission company. No rights-of-way purchases. No holes to dig. Just cable to sow and significant profits to be reaped. In 1995 management decided to sell this piece of its business for $2 billion and a commitment to stay out of it for three years. It returned to being a natural gas transporter, albeit a much richer one. Meanwhile, management monitored the Internet-driven evolution of the telecommunication market. When the three-year restriction was up, Williams announced that it was investing in new business data transmission technologies and returning to the telecommunication wars.

What business are watchmakers in? That is, what do watchmakers sell, whatever they may manufacture? For Rolex, the answer used to be highly accurate timepieces whose quality and price were linked to their sturdiness and precision. When the Japanese flooded the market with cheap, highly accurate digital quartz watches, a technology actually developed in the Swiss watch industry but spurned by it, many Swiss watch companies collapsed. Rolex, however, responded by redefining itself as a jewelry company, selling beauty and prestige in place of timekeeping. It is safe to say that no one today buys a Rolex because they need to know what time it is; but they keep buying extremely expensive ornamental Rolexes at prices whose upper range is $10,000 to $30,000.

At the same time, Swatch, also a Swiss company, saw a different opportunity in this redefinition of watchmaker: it created inexpensive fashion items that also told time. As a fashion item company, Swatch produces hundreds of constantly changing color, pattern, and texture variations on this underlying theme. Its customers typically own several Swatches, each coordinated with the different apparel with which they will be worn. Not a traditional concern of Swiss watchmakers!

What business is an automobile company in? Many people are surprised to learn that the answer does not include much manufacturing. So-called auto manufacturers such as the American Big Three are preeminently designers, assemblers, and marketers of vehicles, including financers of vehicle purchases to dealers, fleet buyers, and consumers. (Add maintenance and upgrade services, and Boeing plays a similar role in aircraft "manufacture." Boeing manufactures only about 30 percent of the parts content of the 777, for example.) Through its Delphi auto parts division, GM manufactures a little over 50 percent of the parts in its cars and trucks. Ford manufactures less than 40 percent, Chrysler less than 30 percent, and BMW barely 10 percent.

In a truck assembly plant in Brazil, Volkswagen is testing a more radical answer to the question of the business it is in. Volkswagen does no manufacturing at all in or for that plant, and no vehicle assembly work either! Vehicle assembly is done by a small group of supersuppliers, each with a supplier network of its own that delivers parts to the assembly plant on a just-in-time basis. Workers employed not by Volkswagen but by the supersuppliers assemble the parts into subassemblies that are attached to the bare vehicle chassis as it moves down the line. What does Volkswagen do? Design, production scheduling, quality control, sales and marketing, financial services. Each vehicle is built to order only, and no one is paid for their work on a vehicle until it has passed inspection and been delivered to the customer who ordered it.

Will this redefinition of Volkswagen's business work? Can it be extended to automobile assembly? Will it lead to production to order of the roughly fourteen million cars and light trucks sold annually in the United States, thereby fulfilling early 1990s visions of a three-day car: three days from customer order to production to delivery? Whether it does or not, there is ample evidence that the automotive industry is on the threshold of a major transformation.

What business are car dealers in? Car dealerships are in the process of being redefined, voluntarily and involuntarily, as customers use the

Internet to order cars, dealers to sell them, and the manufacturers to market them. New car sales as a percentage of dealership profits have dropped sharply. A Chrysler dealer in the tiny town of Kellogg, Idaho, population twenty-six hundred, sold four thousand vehicles in 1997. Auto sales brokered by just one Internet-based car buying service, Auto-by-Tel, have soared past the $1 billion a year mark. More and more people are using Internet services to arrive at a lowest price for the vehicle they want, configured as they want, with the name in hand of a dealer somewhere who will sell it to them at that price. They then ask a local dealer to match that price, threatening to buy through a buying service or the Internet if they do not.

Auto-by-Tel has already stopped signing up dealers, claiming that the twenty-seven hundred currently enrolled are more than enough to serve the country. (At the end of 1997, there were over twenty-one thousand new car dealers in the United States.) With as much as 20 percent of the sales price of a car reflecting postproduction costs—marketing, shipping, dealer inventory, dealer overhead, and profits—that is probably the single greatest opportunity for manufacturers to cut prices and increase their own profits. To do so will require redefining the distribution system that has been in place for almost a century. Not to do so is to ignore the primary imperative of agility: to move from selling products to selling solutions. If you were a car dealer, would you laugh now at the question, "What business are you *really* in?"

Even in the short time that it has been subjected to market forces, health care has witnessed the kinds of opportunities that can come from rethinking what business a company ought to be in. Before his fall from grace, Richard Scott had begun to reposition Columbia/HCA, which had grown to giant proportions on the back of an innovative reconceptualization of profit opportunities in hospital services. Scott had decided to move Columbia/HCA away from growth through facilities acquisition to growth through medical data products. Projecting the acceptance and spread of disease management methodologies, Scott planned on building massive medical databases whose information could be packaged and sold in virtually unlimited variations.

What are the lessons that health care organizations need to learn about rethinking the businesses that they already are, or should, or could be, in from these industrial organization anecdotes?

Perpetual Solution Creation

Agility poses the challenge of responding to a marketplace that expects and rewards a continuing stream of new variations on current solutions and the regular introduction of new kinds of solutions—ones that create whole new markets. The former response is illustrated by the enormous variety of product models that companies offer—credit cards, benefits packages, banking and brokerage accounts, computers, cellular telephones, point-and-shoot cameras—and by the rate at which they are replaced by newer ones, commonly six weeks to three months later. The latter response is illustrated by such market-creating moves as moving from desktop computers to laptops to palmtops, from bulky phones to cellular ones, from selling the telephones to selling the service and giving the telephones away, from broadcast to cable to satellite TV, from private corporate computer networks to Internet-based intra- and extranets.

Continuous improvement of a company's current products and processes is a valuable organizational attribute, but it is not enough to remain competitive for long, however excellent those products and processes may be. The reality is that everyone's marketplace is constantly being destabilized by innovative competitors. Working "smarter, faster, cheaper, and better" improves a company's performance only if it is working on the right thing, and today even the right thing is right only for a little while. Recognizing this, and incorporating it into an organization's operations, challenges prevailing notions of efficiency and quality.

The time taken to optimize operations in terms of traditional, internal financial metrics is too long, and the resources required are no longer justified by the impact of optimization on the company's bottom line. Getting to market *fast*, and if at all possible *first*, with solutions that work well enough for customers to want them and to be able to use them is more important than operational efficiency or getting the quality higher than it needs to be for the solution to be usable. The nature of a solution is such that once it is adopted, the relationship with the customer will provide an economic basis for improvement and further development. Unlike a standard product or service, it is much more painful to a customer to have to replace a solution, especially an individualized solution, than a toaster or an automobile. In some ideal sense, it would be wonderful if software products were bug free upon release. In fact, although they complain vocally, buyers reward the release of new software sooner with bugs than later without them. Similarly, customers have been rewarding Chrysler since the early 1990s for the style of its vehicles and its marketing, in spite of evidence that its vehicle quality is not as high as the competition's.

Every market is different, but to pursue internal goals of efficiency and quality blindly is to be out of touch with marketplace reality. The constantly reexamined strategic goal of an agile organization's management is to optimize organizational responsiveness to a rapidly and unpredictably changing marketplace. Improving production, purchasing, billing, inventory management, logistics, and other business components as individual business processes is important, but as a set of tactics that must be subordinated to an overriding strategy. What must be optimized is the ability to respond to marketplace changes that management identifies as offering the greatest opportunities for growth and profit. To be able to do that requires, along with controlling process costs, a competency in anticipating the potential impact of changes along with a competency in quickly configuring the human and physical resources necessary to exploit the most promising opportunities.

In effect, agility demands competency in managing an organization from the outside—from the marketplace—in. That may be a daunting challenge for people still rooted in the mass production–era business paradigm, which rewarded managing from the inside out, but it is pivotal to organizational success.

Constant Self-Interrogation

Agility challenges managers to examine and constantly reexamine if the organization's policies and personnel are focused on solving the right problems, for customers and for the organization itself. The dynamism of customer relationships means that the most valuable customers today may not be the most valuable customers in three years, or even three months. Who will the best customers be then? What will they value that you have to be able to provide if you are to keep them as customers?

Digital Equipment Corporation has a division that manufactures ATMs and printing equipment for banks. The market, especially in Asia, is growing, but the competition from rival manufacturers is fierce and profit margins are low. In an echo of the Steelcase and IBM strategies, DEC discovered that its best customers were not those who bought the most hardware, but those who needed help designing branch offices, installing the equipment bought from DEC as well as other suppliers, and training the staff at each branch in how to use, maintain, and service that equipment.

To exploit these opportunities for attracting new customers and holding on to what were now perceived as its most valuable customers, changes were instituted. New training and evaluation and reward metrics were required for the sales force. New resources needed to be developed that showed customers the full spectrum of the products and services that DEC was prepared to provide. Furthermore, the target audience now was not only technically knowledgeable equipment purchasing agents, but nontechnical managerial and operational personnel, including branch managers and tellers.

Having identified opportunities for new kinds of solutions, how those solutions should be produced is a question with many more possible answers today than when a company sold products. You can develop, produce, and market the solution yourself, in which case you have all the costs and take all the risks but get to keep all the profits. You can form alliances with other companies, which distributes the risk, lowers the costs, and may shorten development time, but you will have to share the profits. Faced with the need to make choices like this routinely and quickly—recall that solutions target rapidly changing niche markets—new kinds of decision support competencies become invaluable: the ability to estimate time to market accurately; the value of being first and the cost of being late; the risk of guessing wrong; the ability to identify appropriate, trustworthy allies, quickly form working relationships with them, and dissolve these relationships amicably as a solution evolves in ways that either require other allies or its withdrawal from the market; the ability to put a value on changing contributions by partners and to share knowledge openly without hemorrhaging intellectual property.

Alliances are far more valuable in an agile competitive environment keyed to speed and solutions than in the mass production–dominated competitive environment, but as with so much in life, the benefits come at a price. Working collaboratively today requires a commitment to integrating information flow among collaborators in order to integrate business systems and production processes. This requires incorporating into investment in information technology support for standards that allow that kind of integration to take place. Collaboration can transfer new knowledge into your organization, but it will also transfer proprietary knowledge *out*: if you do not have knowledge to offer, you are not likely to be a valued collaborator.

Companies continue to invest in information technology at an increasing rate, but they are not always clear about their objectives. Typically they invest tactically, upgrading performance and adding applications as needed, rather than strategically, to support enterprise-level goals of agility. The same problem affects reengineering initiatives undertaken by companies, the implementation of teaming and empowerment, and developing interactive relationships with customers and suppliers. The objective should not be cutting costs, but creating bases for growth by acquiring new capabilities and competencies that are valued highly by current markets.

To be successful today and tomorrow, an organization, any organization, from educational institution to chip manufacturer, from solo medical practice to global pharmaceutical company, must be able to compete on the basis of cost and value concurrently. That may sound paradoxical on reflection, or even impossible, but it is true.

Competing on cost typically is associated with optimizing recurring processes. Competing on value typically is associated with serving customers for whom cost is not the primary consideration. In an agile environment, in which competition is based on speed and individualized solutions, the premium commanded by new value is short-lived at best. Customers expect new value and know that competition will drive costs down very quickly. Unless they are strongly motivated to be what marketers call "early adopters" or have compelling time constraints, customers discount the new value premium.

Customers have learned to do this because solutions tend to be knowledge-intensive creations. As with designer clothes, it is easy and cheap to copy them. The hard part is coming up with the idea for new combinations of goods, information, and services. The market research, the design and the development, and the marketing eat up time and resources. Once a new solution is released and is successful, imitation of it is virtually guaranteed, and the imitators can set prices that reflect only production costs. They do not have to recoup the research, design, and development costs or the expense of opening up the new market.

Anticipating imitation by competitors, management in agile organizations bases allocations of resources on a constantly changing balance between cost-based process efficiency and cost-intensive new solution creation activities. Followers in an agile environment do not have the advantage over pioneers that they used to have. Today, first to market frequently creates the basis for dominating the market and for reaping the lion's share of the profits. Hewlett-Packard continues to dominate the market for ink-jet and laser printers in large measure because of its ability to manipulate this balance to its advantage. It has for years maintained a bold strategy of bringing out a continuing stream of new models whose price decreases within months to less than half its original price as the next model is introduced.

Having been first into this market, Hewlett-Packard has been able to fend off intense competition from Canon, Epson, and Lexmark, among others, whose new models must be price competitive with the most recently discounted Hewlett-Packard model. Meanwhile, Hewlett-Packard, which buys the engine of its printers—the print mechanism but not the nozzle and its controlling software—from rival Canon, derives very large profits not from the printers themselves, but from selling replacement cartridges and toner!

Managing Knowledge

Agility poses the challenge of managing knowledge as an organization's core asset. This is far more difficult than it sounds. Very few organizations, even those explicitly in the knowledge business such as consultants and universities, have functional knowledge capture and management processes. Making evolving health care knowledge more accessible to more people who can apply it to create health care solutions underlies the Emory University–led consortium referred to earlier, as well as the joint Shared Medical Systems–Crozer Keystone Hospital creation of the Physicians Office of the Future. In Chapter Seven, Leanne Kaiser Carlson and Scott Hendrickson describe the opportunities for leveraging health care information offered by new computer and telecommunication technologies. In Chapter Three, Michael Barton describes a practice management model that leverages back-office organization competency to offer rural consumers higher-quality health care solutions at lower cost.

The norm, unfortunately, is that the overwhelming majority of organizations are critically dependent on what management consultant Alec Lengyel calls "tribal knowledge": the tacit, undocumented knowledge that competent people employ to get their jobs done. Lengyel tells a story from his own experience to illustrate the point.

The tail section of the Boeing 747 is manufactured in Texas to strict Boeing specifications by the LTV Corporation. Originally, the tail was "dry," that is, it did not carry fuel, but it was designed to be "wet" should the need for carrying extra fuel arise, and it was to be built to wet specifications. For several years, LTV-manufactured tails passed inspection and testing without problems, including a test for carrying fuel without leaking. Came the day when Boeing started to implement the capability to carry fuel. Suddenly an unacceptably high percentage of tail sections failed the wetness test and required rework. An initial investigation revealed that the welders were following required procedures exactly as specified in the rule book. Frustrated, Boeing sent in a team of consultants, Lengyel among them, who uncovered the problem and its solution. The first generation of welders were German craftsmen brought in to make sure that this delicate and demanding work was done properly. By the time Boeing used the wet tail capability, the Germans had been replaced by American welders who were trained by the book and who followed the book. The "tribe" of German welders, however, knew enough to know that the book was not completely right to achieve the level of containment required. With their departure, the knowledge of what they actually did left with them.

Capturing tribal knowledge is one critical process in an organization committed to managing knowledge as its core asset. In addition, processes must be put in place for identifying and acquiring relevant new knowledge in the face of rapidly and unpredictably changing market opportunities; organizing this knowledge so that people can access relevant subsets of it quickly and efficiently; and distributing the right knowledge in real time to the right people so that they can use it. Finally, unless people throughout the organization are motivated to create value for the organization and its customers by using knowledge innovatively, knowledge management processes will not improve an organization's competitiveness.

Effective knowledge management thus entails unswerving commitment to putting in place a supportive organizational infrastructure. Personnel recruiting, reward, and evaluation must reflect the value placed on continuous learning and using knowledge to create value. The organization must implement an open information and communication environment, overcoming the security and labor-management relationship problems this raises. A knowledge-driven enterprise must have an adaptive information system, one that learns from the way it is used and changes itself accordingly, and it must be knowledge based. Most, if not virtually all, corporate information systems today remain largely data based, understanding information to be organized data and knowledge to be interpreted information.

It is encouraging that so many companies—over 20 percent of the Fortune 1000 by mid–1997—have created the position of chief knowledge officer to implement effective information and knowledge management processes. But the position can be effective only if knowledge management is made central to strategic planning and the organization of work.

Motivating the Entire Workforce

Agility compels management to put substance into the usually hollow claim that people are an organization's most important asset. Only people can create solutions by using knowledge innovatively. Only people can create the trust that makes collaboration, within and among organizations, possible. Only people can create the trust and mutual understanding necessary to build value-generating networks based on win-win relationships.

Only people *can* do these things. The question remains, *will* they?

Agility is at the opposite pole from the theory of scientific management that dominated early twentieth-century organizational theory. At the start of the newly created industrial corporation, Frederick Winslow Taylor imagined an optimal form for its operation. All knowledge, all expertise, all decision making was to be centralized in the corporate planning department. There was *one right way* to perform each of the many discrete jobs into which the total work of the corporation was to be divided, and only experts, trained as he was in scientific engineering, knew how to divide up the work and how to do each job best. Theirs and theirs alone was the active role.

Taylor's scientific management was transmuted into the management science that remains the core curriculum of virtually all business schools today. His legacy is a managerial philosophy keyed to control, an organizational model keyed to centralized authority, and an operational workforce that ideally does what it is told to do and *only* what it is told to do. Hardly a prescription for creating a think-like-an-owner employee mentality.

Marketplace changes—in the value of speed, knowledge, and solutions—have made the central ideas of management science, no less than of scientific management, increasingly dysfunctional. Where control mandates rigid organizational structures, an agile commercial environment mandates organizational flexibility. Centralized authority must give way to (coordinated) distributed decision making. Centralized expertise must give way to the ability to leverage the knowledge of the entire workforce in order to create a continuous stream of solutions and bring them to market quickly. Control itself must give way to motivation and support as management's primary responsibility.

From the side of management, accountability cannot be restricted to shareholders alone. It must be extended to the workforce as valid stakeholders in the success of the organization. From the side of the workforce, accountability is not management's problem only; it is theirs as well because they are stakeholders in the organization's success.

The agile workplace has the following characteristics:

- A core management competency in motivating an entrepreneurial workforce
- Support for pervasive cooperative relationships, across the organization and with other organizations (for example, suppliers, customers, and partners)
- Deeply distributed authority with strategically coordinated decentralized decision making
- Knowledge- and information-driven operations, supported by an open information and communication environment
- Universal accountability for the organization's success
- Continuous education and training in support of continuously evolving workforce competency requirements to respond to new market opportunities
- Shared responsibility between management and employees for job security in the face of constantly changing markets

Attributes of an Agile Health Care Organization

The temptation is very strong to evade fundamental change in favor of incremental improvement of the status quo: doing better what an organization is currently doing, refining how it is doing it, improving the productivity of who does it. This misses the power of the agility model to effect major improvement by transforming the status quo: working differently in order to produce different things for different markets.

To be competitive in industry today demands more than efficiency, flexibility, and rapid response. Improving quality, cutting costs, and empowering employees are valuable tactics, but they will not by themselves solve any company's problems for long. Such tactics may work in the short run, but they are the modern-day analogue of smarter-faster-cheaper-better ways to manufacture propeller-driven passenger planes after jet-engined planes have been introduced, or improving the quality and lowering the price of portable typewriters after the marketplace has embraced word processing. And what is true for industrial corporations is equally true for health care organizations.

What is demanded even of health care organizations by today's commercial reality is a shift to a new system keyed to continually changing marketplace opportunities and continually escalating customer demands. By whatever name it is characterized—we favor *agility*—this system requires that the employees of an organization work together with one another and with customers, suppliers, partners, and even competitors to produce a constantly changing mix of customer-centered solutions. This may sound like a call to return to the old craft method of production. Craft methods, however, allowed a business to satisfy only a very few customers at a time, and at a premium price; new technologies, especially new information technologies, now allow companies to satisfy the unique requirements of many individual customers at a cost comparable to mass production–era costs, while maintaining high overall volumes of production.

The objective for health care organizations is to use technology to function routinely and cost-effectively in a manner analogous to a hospital's emergency room: responding in an integrated way, on demand, to the full spectrum of an individual customer's requirements by using an appropriate mix of competencies and facilities, near at hand and distributed.

Rather than continuing to function as more efficient stand-alone entities, businesses pursuing agility today are forging collaborative relationships with suppliers, customers, and even competitors, in the process creating extended value-adding production networks. Health care organizations too must create networks for the production of health care solutions, rather than discrete products and services, by developing innovative collaborative relationships with one another. In Chapters Four and Five, Michael Annison, and Rick Gilkey and Gary Lieberman, respectively, discuss the forces driving inter-enterprise cooperation in health care and the distinctive leadership required for effective cooperation.

In recent years, most U.S. companies, including many health care enterprises, have undertaken one or more programs of Total Quality Management, employee empowerment, just-in-time logistics supply, reduced cycle time, and more. Yet many of these companies have seen little sustained bottom-line return for the investments they have made. Often the reason is that these programs, which are tactical responses to marketplace pressures, have been adopted as ends rather than as the means that they in fact are. They are elements of what ought to be a coordinated strategic response to the company's total competitive environment. Agility is precisely such a strategic response.

Because it looks at what *new* things organizations *ought* to be doing, not just at how they can do a better job of what they already are doing, and because it approaches the production of solutions as an integrated system, an agility-based strategic plan challenges the prevailing paradigms of organization, management, production, and competitiveness. It takes no established practices for granted and demands that the processes that support the creation, production, and distribution of goods and services be centered on the customer-perceived value of products and services.

Agility thus requires knowing a great deal about each individual customer and the status of all of the nodes in the production network required to satisfy that customer's requirements. Under the agility model, hospitals, insurers, laboratories, suppliers of drugs, equipment, supplies, or services, physicians, or therapists cannot settle for monitoring their own performance. If they are nodes in a network producing a solution for an individual customer, then they need to be concerned with the performance of the other nodes just as much as their own.

In an agile competitive environment, there is no one right way to organize and operate a company. Management must be able to adopt the mix of multiple and concurrent organizational and operational tactics that will be most effective for that company, given the variety of customers it serves and their evolving requirements. If this is true for GE and IBM, and it is, then it is true for health care organizations as well. The organization of the inherited health care system, put into place between the two world wars, has been strained by changing market requirements beyond its ability to function satisfactorily. It would be a mistake to attempt to replace it by identifying a new structure better suited to today's health care demands. Inevitably that structure would be overwhelmed by tomorrow's different requirements. The right course is to create health care organizations able to configure and reconfigure human, information, and physical resources routinely in response to changing opportunities. To an organization capable of such agility, marketplace change is experienced as new opportunities, not as new requirements threatening the status quo.

To thrive in such a continually evolving environment, an organization must have the right core competencies with which to create new customer opportunities, as well as the competencies to respond to new customer opportunities that present themselves, and unpredictably. And it must be able to move from concept to cash flow in a fraction of the time it now takes, because of the intensity of competition and the rapidity of marketplace change. Doing this demands more than flexible production, whether of goods or services, operational efficiency, or rapid response time. An agile organization must be able to synthesize new productive capabilities quickly. As a result, it is increasingly advantageous for companies to develop new products and services cooperatively with other companies, including direct competitors.

To become agile, then, and to be a valued partner in an evolving market-driven network of win-win inter-enterprise relationships, an organization must possess four strategic capabilities: sell solutions rather than traditional products or services; work collaboratively with other organizations to create, produce, sell, and support solutions; have an adaptive internal organization that supports collaborative relationships by configuring human, capital, and physical resources on demand; and treat people, information, and knowledge as the source of the organization's competitive advantage. The resource allocation priority within these capabilities, and the balance to be struck among them, will be different for different organizations. They will even change over time for the same organization as its market opportunities change. Understanding these capabilities and their interrelationships is the key to developing a migration strategy to agility; continually reassessing them is the key to sustaining agility in the face of competitive pressures, and the tendency of all organizations to see change as a threat.

The chapters that follow reflect movement in the health care industry toward acquiring these capabilities. They reveal that suppliers, providers, payers, and educators of future health care professionals are beginning to make these four capabilities primary strategic objectives.

Selling Solutions

Customers perceive the "products" of an agile organization as solutions to their individual problems. The goal is strategic relationships with customers: long-term relationships that can survive rapid marketplace change. The means for accomplishing this goal are evolving multidimensional solutions—variable individualized combinations of goods, information, and services—that address, and ideally anticipate, customers' problems.

In Chapter Two Martin Raber and Martyn Howgill of the M. D. Anderson Cancer Center in Houston describe a solution-based approach to cancer treatment. The customers here are not only the patients, on whom care delivery is centered, but all of the stakeholders in the solution: insurers, the hospital, referring primary care physicians, and the full range of care providers, from oncology specialists to therapists. The goal of the Cancer Manager model they describe is to respond to the common interests of all of these stakeholders.

In Chapter Three, Michael Barton, CEO of PriCare, describes a practice management model optimized to small, rural health care markets. The model is a solution because it creates win-win relationships in which mutual benefit derives from using information and services collaboratively to serve health care consumers better.

Collaborative Operations

Cooperation—internal and with other companies—is an agile competitor's operational strategy of first choice. The goal is bringing the right products to market as rapidly and as cost-effectively as possible. One strategy for achieving this goal is drawing on existing production resources, from design through field service, regardless of where they are located or who owns them. Intra- and inter-enterprise cross-functional teams, empowerment, reengineering of business processes, virtual companies, and opportunistic partnering, even with direct competitors, are all used to leverage distributed resources to create new solution-products through cooperation. This allows everyone to build on their core competencies, to leverage those world-class human and technological resources that are best suited to new initiatives. Alliances among companies with complementary resources and expertise can reduce sunk costs and risk while concurrently reducing development time, increasing the probability of success, and creating interdependencies on which to build future collaborations.

One of the many forms that cooperation can take is the virtual organization, an opportunistic alliance of core competencies distributed among a number of distinct operating entities, either within a single large organization or among a number of collaborating companies. Carol Graham discusses virtual organizations in detail in Chapter Nine, with an example of a virtual health care organization in Philadelphia. The Visa credit card is a familiar, if largely unappreciated, virtual organization. Today more and more companies, across all industry sectors, from PC assemblers like Dell and Gateway to bicycle vendors, are successfully exploiting the virtual organization model.

Bicycle vendors create finished bicycles by selecting from an enormous variety of specialty components manufactured by companies located around the world. Like the PC assemblers, they benefit from the carefully planned plug-and-play compatibility of these components, which allows the system integrator to exploit rapidly evolving technology and volatile pricing to optimize the performance and price of the systems they integrate for customers. At the other end of the consumer product spectrum, Dell Computer does precisely the same thing, and with such success that its larger and far richer rival, Compaq, is emulating its production strategy. As a network of affiliated physicians, staff and private, available on demand, each clinical "service" in a hospital is a kind of virtual organization. A more innovative approach might involve pooling clinical, laboratory, and research resources among a group of competing hospitals in a single metropolitan area.

In Chapter Four, Michael Annison, president of the Westrend Group, describes how health care organizations are beginning to use cooperation as a competitive weapon and what will be required if they are to cooperate more intensively.

In Chapter Five, Emory University professors Roderick Gilkey and Gary Lieberman discuss the distinctive leadership challenges that must be overcome if organizations are to create mutually beneficial cooperative working relationships.

Adaptive Organization

Agile organizations thrive on change and uncertainty. Their flexible structure permits rapid reconfiguration of human and physical resources. They can support multiple, concurrent organizational configurations keyed to the requirements of different market opportunities. They are designed to optimize their ability to exploit rapidly and unpredictably changing opportunities for information and services-rich, high-value-added, short-market-lifetime products. For each different opportunity, management can answer differently the question, "What is the best way for us to be organized?" Internal teams, inter-enterprise teams, peer collaborations, hierarchical collaborations, lattice structures, and flattened pyramids have applications that are appropriate to achieving a particular project's ends.

In Chapter Six, James Cramer and Wendy Lyons of Scottsdale Health Care describe how their organization responded to new market opportunities—reflecting changing demographics and new kinds of health care services—and new customer challenges, reflecting more knowledgeable and more demanding consumers.

Leveraging People, Information, and Knowledge

People and information differentiate competitors in the world of agile competition. What an organization sells is its ability to convert the knowledge, skills, and information embodied in its personnel into solution products for individual customers. What a company's most valuable customers are really paying for is access to people who are capable of synthesizing solutions to their problems out of the knowledge they possess and the information and production technologies the company makes available to them. The first task of an agile competitor is to create a communication and information environment that leverages the impact of people and knowledge on its bottom line. A surprisingly large number of companies lack a systematic inventory of the expertise their employees possess, the expertise the organization will need to move into new markets, and a plan for moving from the first state to the second. Recognition of this ignorance underlies the growing interest in core competency inventories, knowledge capture processes, and innovative education and training programs.

In Chapter Seven, Leanne Kaiser Carlson and Scott Hendrickson of the Kaiser Technology Group describe new and emerging health care information "products" that are being made possible by information technologies.

In Chapter Eight, Morton Sosland and David Nash of Thomas Jefferson University and Medical College discuss the changes in medical education that will be required to produce physicians adapted to an agile health care system. They describe as well a series of initiatives that illustrate unambiguously that a number of medical schools around the country are collaborating with payer organizations and vendors to implement those curricular changes.

In the concluding chapter, Carol Graham of the Agility Forum provides a simple self-assessment tool, keyed to these four organizational capabilities, for developing a migration strategy to agility. The series of exercises she describes, linked to worksheets she provides, lead from prioritizing the market forces driving an organization to change its status quo, through prioritizing those attributes of an agile organization that would be most valuable to it, to outlining an action plan for acquiring those selected attributes.

Conclusion

The current business environment is causing health care organizations at all levels to reinvent agility, and they are doing so piecemeal, as industry initially did: a solution initiative here and a collaboration initiative there; an innovative information technology application in one hospital, a reorganization of the workforce in another. Seeing agility in a comprehensive context challenges health care organizations to shift from learning exclusively from their own experience to adapting to their distinctive needs a systematic solution to a strongly similar problem already developed by others.

Fundamental health care system change is inescapable; becoming agile is inevitable. The short-term option of substituting for fundamental change improving the efficiency of current operations is denial of reality. For better and for worse, there is a new reality in health care. At all levels it is subject to prevailing market forces. Health care remains different from other services, but it is no longer different enough to ignore the commercial sector of the economy.

One commercial sector lesson that health care organizations must learn is the value for them of agility as a model for change.

Agility is as relevant to public and private services companies and institutions, for profit and not for profit, as to the industrial corporations in which it first emerged. Health care professionals need to familiarize themselves with agility because, like it or not, the economy is assimilating the characteristics and the values of agility, as one hundred years ago it assimilated the characteristics and the values of the then newly invented industrial corporation. Agility-based competition and the mass production–based competition that preceded it are like two different games, each with its own rules for playing and its own strategies for winning.

The question is not which game is better but which game is being played. The answer is clear: agility is the game that the most successful companies are playing today. To compete in today's marketplace, players and coaches have to learn the rules of the new game and the strategies favorable to success.

2

An Integrated Disease Management Model

Martin N. Raber, Martyn W. C. Howgill

Unlike the episodic nature of most interactions with the health care delivery system in the United States, cancer care is a life-long engagement. Once diagnosed, a cancer patient faces a battle for survival, followed by a lifetime of consequences. Unfortunately, all too many patients become involved in an episodically oriented system that views them as appointments filling a schedule, tests in line to be reviewed, and treatments waiting to be given.

This fragmentation of cancer diagnosis, treatment, and follow-up care has implications not only for patients but also for payers. Due to the complexity of the disease, managed care companies have difficulty coordinating multidisciplinary care, authorizing appropriate care plans, and denying inappropriate treatments and diagnostic tests. Improved outcomes, including significant savings, can be realized when the patient is accurately diagnosed and provided the appropriate treatment plan early in the disease process. In addition, expert management is required at critical points throughout the course of the disease, which can result in further outcome improvements.

The needs and expectations of patients and health plan enrollees have come to be seen as conflicting with those of payers—be they self-insured employers, managed care companies, or risk-holding physicians. The University of Texas M. D. Anderson Cancer Center's challenge has been to find a strategic solution to reconciling this conflict that meets the needs of all its customers without sacrificing the interests of any. It has attempted to take a holistic view of treatment and seeks to provide not only an improved chance for survival and a better quality of life for patients, but also to produce for payers and risk-holding physicians the most effective use of premium dollars.

M. D. Anderson's model for cancer management is a comprehensive disease management program based on the research, expertise, and knowledge of the center's faculty and on market understanding of payers' requirements. The faculty has developed computerized, multidisciplinary guidelines for the continuum of cancer care that address cancer prevention recommendations, the workup of patients suspected of having cancer, the evaluation and treatment of patients with cancer, and follow-up care after treatment.

Together with detailed care plans, this information has been used to develop a series of products—treatment oversight, specialized cancer case and utilization management, capitated payment methods, and quality, cost, and outcomes analyses—that allow better organization and oversight of care delivery and address the appropriate use of clinical trials and other specialized services. Through integration with provider networks, insurance companies, and large, self-insured employers, M. D. Anderson's aim has been to provide better organized, less costly cancer care with more predictable and continuously improving outcomes.

This chapter describes Cancer Manager,™ a project that highlights three facets of organizational agility and attempts to integrate into a patient-centered solution what had been a group of discrete, expertise-centered, medical services. In doing so, the Anderson Center reexamined who its customers were, incorporating into the planning for and the benefits from the new integrated cancer care solution a broader range of internal and external stakeholders in that care than just the patient. Finally, it has begun to use information technology to create a shared knowledge base that can improve quality and lower costs.

Health Care Reform

In responding to their marketplaces, health care organizations inevitably have had to address the impact of almost two decades of efforts to redesign the delivery system and reduce its growing burden on the nation's economy. Reform has been highlighted by two major developments. First came the introduction of Medicare's prospective payment system in the early 1980s and the subsequent and continued reduction by federal policymakers of Medicare reimbursement levels. Second was the rapid penetration in many markets of managed care models in their various forms. As a consequence and in order to succeed, health care providers have had to respond with agility and entrepreneurial action to meet their missions and their margins.

In the face of such stress, some community institutions have turned to for-profit saviors to inject capital and management expertise. As a result, we have witnessed the aggressive tactics of Wall Street juggernauts like Hospital Corporation of America, its successor Columbia/HCA, Tenet Health Care, health maintenance organizations too numerous to mention, and many others that approach treatment of the sick and injured as a profit-producing venture.

This rapid growth of proprietary health care has added to the pressures on the nonprofit and public sector providers. Employers and insurance companies, which understand and respect the management discipline required to meet quarterly earnings expectations of stockholders, have used to their own advantage the downward price pressures represented by the for-profit hospitals' success at streamlining their operations. Proprietary health care has helped set new standards for what can be achieved on a cost per unit of care delivered.

Less efficient providers, absent the discipline of the profit motive, have inadvertently contributed to proprietary margins by enabling them to maintain reimbursement schedules that produce unusually high margins. This is no more than the result of the marketplace at work. The range of market pricing for health care has limited elasticity. For-profit providers can charge at the market rates that their nonprofit and public sector competitors must sustain in order to cover the latter's inefficiencies. What is more, because the supply of for-profit beds and facilities is limited, especially at the tertiary and quaternary service levels, most large health plans and employers are virtually forced to include less efficient providers on their rosters. But while doing so, through such practices as competitive bidding, they certainly have brought significant pressure to bear on all providers to maximize their efficiency.

Over the past fifteen years, these efforts to contain costs have taken various forms. Delivery system management has shifted its focus from cost cutting, principally evidenced by widespread layoffs and huge purchasing consortia, to more sophisticated efforts that have embraced the management principles of gurus like W. Edwards Deming, Joseph Juran, and Peter Senge. These organizations have sought continuous improvement and learning about how to meet their customers' requirements better, and they have learned to become more agile and competitive.

During this period of turbulent change and health care reform, provider leadership has also responded to market needs, as well as their own need to survive, by forming large, integrated delivery systems. These have linked regionally dispersed physician networks, inpatient and outpatient facilities, various other health care components from home health care to pharmacies, and, in some cases, insurance entities.

Indeed, the management of risk has undergone perhaps the most striking change of any other aspect of health care during these troubled years. Increasingly the risk once borne by the insurance industry, the traditional bearer, is being passed along to providers, who, for a fixed fee per enrollee per month, agree to provide to a defined population the care that is contractually agreed on.

This shift in who bears the risk has been accelerating for two intersecting reasons. First, self-insured employers and large insurance companies have seen their own margins eroded by the increased costs of providing employees with adequate health care.

This is a problem that becomes exacerbated during times of exceptionally low employment, when the competition for labor requires employers to provide an attractive benefits package in order to recruit and retain a workforce.

Second, the provider market has faced a declining inpatient census, the result of declining lengths of stay per hospital visit (triggered by the emergence of the prospective payment system and managed care), and improved clinical treatments that have shifted patients to outpatient settings or have greatly shortened the requirements for them to remain as inpatients.

Together, these two trends have led to the development of mutually beneficial arrangements between the large, self-insured employer, the insurance company, and the provider network. Medicare and Medicaid, as the largest insurance programs in the nation, are contributing to this market shift with the development of their own health maintenance organizations.

Implications for M. D. Anderson Cancer Center

It is in this milieu that M. D. Anderson found itself in the early 1990s confronting its own challenges as a specialty institution. In examining how to respond to these market forces, a number of factors have driven its business development and marketing strategies.

First among these is M. D. Anderson's national and even international reputation among patients and referring physicians, a view reflected in its regular annual ranking by *U.S. News & World Report* as one of the top two cancer care providers in the United States. Proprietary surveys conducted by the Anderson indicate that many patients see it as offering their best hope for survival, especially in cancer cases that community medicine has felt necessary to refer up the medical care hierarchy to specialized centers such as the Anderson.

This reputation influences the Anderson's unusual patient origin distribution, which has been a driving factor in the development of its competitive strategy. Most providers typically attract some 80 percent of their patients from their own and surrounding counties, with 20 percent traveling longer distances. This Pareto principle tends to hold true for even the most prestigious medical centers and clinics, including the Anderson's many sister institutions on the Texas Medical Center campus. However, only 30 percent of M. D. Anderson's patients originate locally. (Another 30 percent come from across Texas, another 30 percent from throughout the United States, and some 10 percent come from around the world.) This patient distribution has provided the Anderson with some insulation against the economic incursions of managed care, which would have been far greater if its local market had represented a more typical 80 percent of its business.

Texas law plays into M. D. Anderson's business development strategy. State statute requires that the Anderson accept all Texans regardless of their ability to pay (unless they have insurance that channels them to another provider). This same law also prohibits accepting patients from outside the state without their demonstrated ability to pay. As a result, M. D. Anderson has felt the impact of managed care and health care principally at the local level, since out-of-state patients tend to be covered by more traditional indemnity insurance plans. Although the local marketplace represents only 30 percent of its business, it nevertheless represents M. D. Anderson's greatest challenge in responding with agility to its local customers' requirements.

For example, among some health care purchasers, M. D. Anderson labors under a reputation as a high-cost, academic, and research-driven center to which only the most severe cases should be referred. Employers and managed care plans have expressed concern that the Anderson is too expensive to include as a provider in their plans for cancers that they believe can be appropriately treated in the local community. The problem with this view is that medicine has yet to devise a means by which it can prospectively differentiate so-called simple cancers from those that will become clinically more complicated. For the newly diagnosed patient, an accurate and precise diagnosis is critically important. For M. D. Anderson, whose mission is to eradicate cancer, its solution has been to develop a product that responds to the needs of its payer market for a cost-effective product while maximizing appropriate accessibility for its patient market.

Success at achieving its mission requires the attraction of patients for at least two purposes. First, although M. D. Anderson is a campus of the University of Texas, it receives only 16 percent of its income from state appropriations; the balance of its revenue must come from patient care, research grants, and philanthropic support. Second, it needs appropriately qualified patients to fill the research protocols through which it improves its ability to fight the more than four hundred different types of cancer so far identified. Indeed, accelerating the cycle times on these research protocols (more than seven hundred are currently active) can accelerate the rate at which these advances are made.

While many general hospitals and academic health centers have responded to this need for patients by becoming part of a local integrated network, the Anderson has not considered this option for several reasons. First, in the commercially insured population, the incidence of cancer is relatively rare (two per thousand per year). M. D. Anderson needs to contract with as many insurers as possible to ensure patient flow. Second, if it were to join a closed network, even a large one, the Anderson would be limiting potential referrals. Third, the Anderson is the sole Texas provider of certain tertiary and quaternary services and must be able to contract with all payers for these cases. Finally, as a state institution and resource, the Anderson believes that it cannot act as an exclusive provider for any payer, insurer, or provider group.

One additional factor influencing this complex picture is that M. D. Anderson operates at virtually full capacity. In the case of some types of cancer, demand for its services are so strong that some patients wait one or two weeks before they are even seen. Although steps are being taken to increase capacity, the compelling challenge for the next decade is to bring to the Anderson those patients best able to benefit from its programs, while leaving to community providers those that can most appropriately be treated there. How best to do this, while meeting both the expectations of patients and the requirements of payers, is at the root of M. D. Anderson's development of a product it has named Cancer Manager.™

Paradigm Shifts and Other Barriers

M. D. Anderson's strategic response to the larger health care environment and its own local market forces has been to apply disease management concepts to the delivery of cancer care for enrolled populations in southeast Texas. To do so, it has been necessary for it to attempt three fundamental paradigm shifts.

First, faculty clinicians have had to change from thinking about individual patients to thinking about populations. This runs counter to physician training, which has focused on the individual whose immediate needs are before them. The Anderson physicians must consider as their patients not only those with symptoms today, but also those who might present tomorrow and those who might be prevented from developing symptoms at all. As well, they need to consider patients with cancer who are unable to come to M. D. Anderson. (In a separate initiative, M. D. Anderson has committed significant resources to a new cancer prevention division that is enjoying significant research and clinical success.)

Second, the traditional cancer treatment model has seen faculty balance a complex relationship with referring physicians, on whom they have historically depended for patients. Texas law, however, which previously required a physician referral to the Anderson, was changed in 1995 to permit patients to self-refer to the institution. But even with this statutory change, some two-thirds of all patients seen at M. D. Anderson arrive after involvement by a referring doctor. These same referring physicians, particularly oncologists and surgeons, continue to play an influential gatekeeping role in controlling and sometimes restricting the flow of patients to the Anderson and are therefore often seen as competitors as well as partners.

In the disease management paradigm, the Anderson sees community physicians as collaborating partners with whom faculty must work in determining who and what is treated where, when, and how. The new focus is on a team approach to the disease process that incorporates community providers as partners and that reduces and even eliminates economic competition.

This attempt to align the community physicians' and M. D. Anderson's financial interests is the third key paradigm shift necessary for a disease management response to market needs. Historically, all the players in the health care system except for providers—employers (and the government), insurers and managed care organizations, and patients—have shared at least one common concern: cost. Each still wants to avoid the risk of financial catastrophe from cancer. The employer needs to fix an amount for employee health benefits and be able to budget annual expenses. The insurers and managed care companies similarly require bottom-line predictability. Even fully insured patients express their worries about what diagnosis and a full course of treatment might cost them.

Providers, however, have only recently become concerned about costs, a concern that began with their assuming the financial risk for care through contractual capitation. A requirement of the disease management model applied to cancer has been to align the financial interests of all players in the system and to fix the risk. This is especially needed if the collaboration between community doctors and the Anderson physicians is to work. Only by sharing risk and working together can these providers reach optimal results from both a clinical and cost standpoint.

Making such paradigm shifts is complicated by M. D. Anderson's status as an academic institution. Faculty enjoy the privileges of academic freedom and tenure, and reaching consensus on such matters has been and remains an important step in the successful introduction of this new initiative. Before sharing their intellectual capital with the community, the Anderson's medical staff had to be convinced that it was to their advantage to do so. Sensitivities on this point run high. The fear is that community providers will simply trade on the M. D. Anderson name without meeting clinical practice and quality requirements. Indeed, providing the appropriate case management and oversight throughout the system is a delicate undertaking that must take into account the egos of all involved.

Finally, a critical barrier that had to be overcome before launching this new product has been the challenge of upgrading and integrating the information systems essential to the program's operational success. Cancer Manager™ is an information-driven model. It must be able to track patients across multiple access points and provide practitioners and managers throughout the community with accurate and complete clinical and financial data on demand. Like many other academic institutions populated by independent and brilliant thinkers, the Anderson's various information systems have grown up as independent islands, with communication among them achieved only with some difficulty.

Although these typically department-based systems met some of the automation needs of their respective areas, the Anderson recognized that it urgently needed to integrate patient-centered data into a repository that would be available across the entire enterprise. This shift in its fundamental information technology strategy began with the creation of an on-line data warehouse that integrated clinical and financial data from many different source application systems, which often resided on disparate technology platforms. Completion of this institutional database was the initial phase of a program that continues with the creation of an institutionwide, computer-based patient record that will enable on-line access to the majority of information currently maintained in the paper record. This initiative will continue with a third and final phase that will integrate transcribed documents, manual documents, images, and externally generated patient-related documents into the same central repository.

Cancer Manager™

The concept of disease management is that it organizes and oversees the treatment of patients throughout the course of their illness. This includes prevention services, diagnosis, treatment, follow-up care, and, if necessary, hospice services. In the traditional cancer care model, there are several challenges. First, it has been difficult to coordinate the multidisciplinary nature of diagnosis and treatment. Second, the expertise to approve or deny care is often lacking. Third, patients, families, and sometimes even referring physicians hold unreasonable outcomes expectations, believing that regardless of disease stage, survival must surely be possible. Last, controlling the high costs of uncoordinated episodes of care has often proved impossible. The promise of the disease management model is that it can improve both the quality and cost of clinical outcomes by starting at suspicion, rather than diagnosis, by focusing on the complete spectrum of cancer care, and by standardizing and coordinating that care.

Cancer Manager™ is a comprehensive disease management program based on M. D. Anderson's knowledge about and continuing research into the prevention, diagnosis, and treatment of cancers of all types. At its core are multidisciplinary guidelines and pathways. Practice guidelines provide an overview of a disease process along with the approaches to multidisciplinary medical care for that process, based on expert consensus of current practice standards. They provide a broad overview across the continuum of cancer management and through a series of care episodes. Collaborative care pathways provide more details about daily, expected events and interventions in a single episode of care within a specific disease process. Care paths define what happens at each decision point of a practice guideline, and both guidelines and pathways, with some restricted access, are accessible using computer software and the Internet to help physicians with diagnostic work-ups, treatment, follow-up, and aftercare services. In addition, prevention guidelines provide standards to community physicians for what screening tests are appropriate and when, for the evaluation of abnormal screening results, and for patient education materials. These education materials have obvious benefits for patients and serve also to decrease the number of unnecessary consults, identify cancers at earlier stages, and reduce the primary care physician's liability for missing a potentially detectable cancer in its earlier stages.

Diagnostic algorithms help educate the primary care physician regarding the initial workup of the patient when cancer is first suspected and establish identifiable trigger points for referral to an appropriate specialist. In addition to benefiting patients, this approach reduces unnecessary testing, a significant problem in the community, and inappropriate, expensive, and time-consuming referrals.

In order to extend its effectiveness in this regard, the Anderson has assembled a network of community physician providers who have agreed to base their own diagnosis and treatment practice on these guidelines and pathways. A roster of services defines the appropriate site for treatment, which can be in the community physician's office or hospital or at M. D. Anderson. Privileges for procedures are based on board certification, experience, facilities, and frequency of performance. Since everyone in the network shares the capitated risk, there is no financial friction to interfere with seeking optimal clinical results for the patient, the employer, and the insurer. Quality and outcome measures are based on benchmarks established within the pathways. Case and utilization management reduce unnecessary procedures and hospital stays based on the guidelines.

An additional benefit for the community practice is the improved management of legal risk. Cancer Manager™ offers community network members the opportunity to reduce their exposure to malpractice suits, if the appropriate guidelines and pathways have been observed, by providing a sound clinical basis for legal support in the courtroom in the event of litigation. In addition, network doctors enjoy the marketing benefits of M. D. Anderson's name, which in Houston are considerable and provide a significant competitive advantage, and their patients gain access to world-class, multidisciplinary cancer care in a convenient community setting.

Within this overarching model are built a series of disease management products to meet the varying needs of different customers. With regard to providing actual cancer care, M. D. Anderson has prepared itself to provide carved-out services by accepting full risk for all cancer patients within a defined population. It has successfully piloted such an approach on a population of thirty thousand Houstonians since 1996 and is about to provide similar services for much larger groups. The Anderson has also developed a comprehensive second opinion program and offers treatment planning where that is all that is required.

Given the great variety of needs in the market, Cancer Manager™ has been deliberately designed for agility. For example, in addition to cancer care itself, the Anderson provides utilization management services and case management support. Further, it provides analytical services around costs, outcomes and quality, and physician profiles of performance, including utilization by provider and disease site, and high-level benchmarking. The benchmarking allows physicians to reduce unwarranted variation in practice patterns and provides them with the opportunity for continuous improvement and learning from the best practices among their peers.

Cancer Manager's business service component includes offering claims adjudication services such as authorization validation, conformation of treatment modalities, and review of comorbid conditions and concurrent treatments. Meanwhile, the degree of financial risk assumed by M. D. Anderson can vary from the full risk assumption of carved-out disease management and care delivery, to no-risk assumption with second opinion and utilization, case management, and analytical services, depending on customer requirements.

The internal infrastructure of Cancer Manager™ has been designed like a mini–health plan. The key components within the institution are member services, health care management, provider relations, network development, sales and marketing, financial and business operations, and third-party administrator and information systems functions. Each area underwent a comprehensive planning and testing process to ensure appropriate delivery of results required by different customer groups. These requirements were identified early in the product development process through market research and qualitative feedback from both internal and external sources.

Although M. D. Anderson is still in the roll-out phase of Cancer Manager,™ the anticipated benefits of the program are many. First, it is expected that the appropriateness of care will be based on evidence and the expertise of M. D. Anderson's internationally recruited faculty. Second, techniques and procedures used in care are monitored for their efficacy and resource consumption, providing a sound basis for their continuous improvement.

For example, in 1996 the Anderson began placing thoracic surgery patients requiring a lobectomy with wedge resection on a clinical path. In the first year, one of two patients was enrolled; in 1997 three of four were. After the first two years, average length of stay has decreased from 7.8 to 6.8 days and is both declining steadily and a half-day lower than those patients remaining off path. Mean costs have shown similar declines and are more than 5 percent lower for pathway patients. These lower costs result in part from a reduction of unnecessary variation in patient treatment, such as the administration of fewer chest X-rays during the patient's stay, a benefit for both patient and payer. Perhaps the greatest benefit is that the readmission rate for pathway patients has declined from 5 to 3 percent during this same period.

A third benefit is benchmarking and physician profiling. This information is available to provide feedback to partners in the delivery system, thereby offering them a basis for maximizing their clinical efficiency and effectiveness. Feedback is critical in enabling physicians to identify best practices and in reassuring payers that they are receiving the best value for their health care dollar. A fourth and critically important benefit of Cancer Manager™ is that it helps reduce the length of time it takes for new cancer diagnostic techniques and therapies to become available to patients in the community setting.

There are other benefits as well, including controlling resource utilization and developing predictability for cancer care costs for an at-risk population. During M. D. Anderson's pilot of Cancer Manager,™ enrollment in the program from September 1996 through August 1997 was thirty thousand. During that time, 1,389 authorizations were given for various procedures, with a denial rate of 7.5 percent. Sixty-nine new patients were identified. The patient-days per thousand for patients treated under Cancer Manager™ were four per thousand; for patients who chose an alternate hospital in the provider network, patient days per thousand were twenty-three—almost six times higher. The expected actuarial standard for oncology patients is ten days per thousand.

Based on these benefits and preliminary results, M. D. Anderson believes that its ability to respond with agility to market requirements is a critical competitive advantage and that Cancer Manager™ is an important means for achieving this goal.

The Future

Implementing an integrated, patient-centered disease management model has taken a considerable investment of time and energy by M. D. Anderson's faculty and staff. It has brought the organization together in new ways to respond to the multiple and diverse requirements of its various markets. This commitment to becoming market driven has produced significant shifts in faculty attitudes toward the most efficacious treatment of cancer and holds promise that the Anderson will be better able to thrive in the ever-increasing competitive and financial challenges of health care delivery. The agility required to develop Cancer Manager™ is a valuable new strength that will stand the institution in good stead for years to come. Even more important, it will enable M. D. Anderson, already an extraordinary place for the diagnosis and treatment of cancer, to better meet the needs of patients and families from across the world who seek the hope that they can survive.

3

Consolidated Rural Health Care

Michael W. Barton

Since the creation of Medicare and Medicaid in the mid–1960s, the U.S. health care system has been in a constant state of change. With so many dollars suddenly available through these new federal and state reimbursement programs, health care became a financially driven industry. The development of for-profit health care companies and alternative health care delivery systems was largely driven by the need to be better positioned to capture third-party health care dollars. At the same time, because of the constant adjustments that were being made to the system—the introduction of diagnosis-related groups (DRGs) and managed care, among others—health care companies whose budgets were keyed to these reimbursement programs found themselves hustling to keep up with these adjustments. Health care managers had to become very agile or risk being shut out of the game.

Contributing to the need for agility has been the changing attitude of private industry. As the Medicare system cut federal reimbursement dollars, providers began to pass the unreimbursed costs on to insured patients. Most of these costs ultimately were paid by private industry through employee health insurance programs, in a move commonly referred to as cost shifting. The shift to managed care, with its continuing pressure on cost and reimbursement, to a large extent has been driven by industry reaction against double-digit inflation of health care costs. Frequent comments by auto industry executives that they have more health care dollars in a car than steel dollars is expressive of this frustration.

This chapter describes an agile entrepreneurial response to a health care opportunity: targeting a neglected niche market. Taking a cue from Wal-Mart, PriCare, Inc. is creating a network of multi-specialty rural medical practices, each co-owned with the practicing physicians, that offer consumers an attractive alternative to traveling to urban or suburban practitioners. By making the physicians stakeholders, PriCare motivates sensitivity to the marketplace and a concern for the patient's perception of the quality of delivered care. By consolidating multiple complementary practices, significant provider savings are realized and the total patient experience is significantly improved: travel time is reduced, scheduling is simplified, and information and testing are centralized. By imposing a common, information-centered practice management model, PriCare has significantly reduced its back-office and overhead costs with no impact on care quality.

The Evolving Health Care Management Mindset

Among the numerous examples of organizations that have felt their way to agile capabilities over the past twenty years, three stand out as particularly illustrative of an evolving agile health care management mind-set: HCA, Health Horizons, and PriCare.

When DRGs were instituted by Medicare, hospital inpatient census volumes dropped dramatically and virtually overnight. The largest for-profit company at that time, HCA, could not sustain its stock value in a public market with patient volumes and revenues falling. In response, HCA's management took the company private through a leveraged buy-out, made the changes necessary to operate at lower census levels, and then took the company public again when revenue growth, costs, and earnings could be sustained under the new system.

DRGs and increased government and private industry concerns about rising costs created an environment conducive to the development of alternative delivery systems, principally in the outpatient area. Outpatient surgery companies, such as Medical Care American and Surgical Care Affiliates, evolved during this period. So did other forms of outpatient specialty companies: Image America, specializing in radiology services, and Rehability, specializing in physical therapy services; Coventry Corporation, a health maintenance organization (HMO); PhyCor, a physician practice management company; and Hospital Management Professionals, a hospital management company. In effect, these companies took traditional integrated hospital-based support departments and packaged them into separate, more cost-effective, and easier-to-access niche service companies.

With the advent of managed care and exclusive contracting between major medical centers and payers, many stand-alone outpatient surgery centers were dismayed at being excluded from contracting. One surgery center company, Health Horizons, responded by selling ownership interest to major medical centers in exchange for access to its managed care contracts. The benefits to the medical center were that it could provide a low-cost surgery alternative to enhance its contracting abilities, it could offload certain types of surgery (such as eye surgery) that can be performed in surgery centers at lower cost, and it improved its relationships with its surgeons. In addition, the surgery center was able to gain access to a larger patient base along with its access to new managed care contracts.

Although President Clinton's attempt in 1993 to pass new national health care legislation was unsuccessful, the mere threat caused more restructuring by providers and payers as they scrambled to reposition themselves in anticipation of future legislation. For-profit health care companies, for example, began consolidating into larger and larger corporations, with the Columbia/HCA system leading the way. The not-for-profit sector then accelerated its own efforts to consolidate and form networks in order to remain competitive with the for-profit companies. Physicians, who ultimately control 80 percent of the health care dollar directly or through the therapies they recommend, began to consolidate their practices and organize their own networks, for example, by combining into multispecialty groups, selling their practices to practice management companies or medical centers, and forming medical services organizations or independent practice associations.

On the payer side, managed care and risk sharing have become increasingly important objectives, often pursued through the formation of alliances. Ultimately, however, there is one common driving force behind these various consolidation efforts: the perceived need to create more compact and less costly health care organizations that are better positioned to secure care contracts.

Health Care in Rural Areas

Urban and suburban health care providers have for some time been feeling the forces driving system-level change, and they have been reacting more or less successfully to the impact of these changes. The result is an increasingly competitive health care system in urban areas. Rural areas, on the other hand, have historically been sheltered from changes in the health care system to a significant degree, in part because of the smaller, highly fragmented markets they represent, in part because of their distinctive demographics. Rural areas do not lend themselves to consolidation primarily because of their small-business orientation.

Rural health care, as with rural retail businesses, is mainly a mom-and-pop operation. The typical physician is a solo practitioner with unsophisticated employees and systems that are frequently managed by the physician's spouse or parent. The bang for the buck has historically not been there for the larger urban health care companies. Additionally, the rural population tends to be spread out. The county seat may have only six thousand people, while the county area has over thirty thousand people. This, too, makes consolidation at a single site more difficult.

For these reasons, rural communities until recently received scant attention from larger-scale providers, which looked to urban areas, with their larger populations and thus larger markets and greater opportunities for both providers and payers. But as competition has increased and more emphasis has been placed on networking and patient referrals, rural areas have begun receiving considerably more attention. For-profit companies such as Columbia/HCA, Community Health Systems, and Hospital Management Associates increasingly are targeting hospitals in rural communities for acquisition or networking.

A good example of this turnaround in attitude is the HCA story. When management took the company private to deal with the impact of DRGs, they spun off many of their rural and small hospitals to Healthtrust. Later, when HCA was acquired by Columbia, Healthtrust was reacquired because of its referral base and its potential impact on Columbia's ability to secure managed care contracts. The not-for-profit hospital industry is being forced to do the same thing; in fact, the not-for-profit providers are matching the for-profit industry in aggressiveness. To some extent, large medical centers are being forced into action as a strategic defensive mechanism: if they do not secure these markets, their competitors will. Both the for-profits and not-for-profits are attempting to acquire or hire primary care physicians in rural communities in order to secure patient referrals and build volume. On the payer side, however, managed care generally is still not a major factor in these communities, although discounted fee-for-service is quite common. Nevertheless, as the larger providers encroach on rural areas, they will bring managed care with them.

One factor that is enabling the extension of recent urban health care changes to rural markets is that the health care system characteristics of rural communities are quite homogeneous throughout the country. Thanks to the Hill-Burton Program created in the

1950s, which provided ready and cheap capital to build hospitals in rural areas, the U.S. countryside is dotted with small rural community hospitals. More often than not, they are county owned, undercapitalized, poorly equipped, and operating with a modest daily patient census, predominantly Medicare and Medicaid patients, which means that a large majority of the hospitals' funding is from government sources. It is also not unusual for the hospital to be receiving a subsidy from the local tax base, which often spells the difference between closing or survival. Furthermore, because of the difficulty of attracting physicians to these rural areas, the community is typically medically underserved, particularly by primary care physicians. The end result is a high out-migration of the more affluent or the more mobile insured population to urban areas for their health care. All of these factors are combining to fragment even more an already badly fragmented health care delivery system in nonurban and rural communities. Although this fragmentation makes consolidation more difficult, therein also lies the opportunity.

Rural Opportunities

The for-profit health care industry in particular has spawned and trained a large number of entrepreneurs who are able to spot health care business opportunities that invariably arise in rapidly changing environments. A good example is the Hospital Affiliates, Inc. (HAI) story.

In 1981, when HAI was acquired by HCA, a number of HAI executives left and subsequently founded several new companies. In fact, at a recent fifteen-year reunion of former HAI executives, an informal survey disclosed that over the preceding fifteen years, this group had founded sixty-six new health care companies, including Medical Care America, American Healthcorp, Republic Health, Champion Health Care, and Community Health Systems. Former HCA executives have also formed new companies. This ability to form new companies has been fostered by the ready availability of venture and investment capital to back experienced health care management teams with sound business plans. Additionally, health care has proved to be a great niche business. The rural market is now offering attractive health care business opportunities for leading-edge agile entrepreneurs and managers, and increasingly is attracting the attention of established as well as start-up companies.

PriCare, Inc., of Brentwood, Tennessee, is one of these emerging companies. In surveying this unique market, the company's founders recognized five demographic factors that begged for consolidation:

- Rural communities suffer considerable out-migration of patients to larger urban areas. It is not unusual for a small community to have as little as a 35 percent to 40 percent market penetration. If this out-migration could be reversed, there would be an enormous favorable economic and service impact to the community.

- The hospitals in these communities are typically undercapitalized and can provide only minimal services. They are ill positioned to provide services needed to reattract patients. It is not unusual to hear remarks such as, "The local hospital is okay, but if you're really sick, you had better not go there." Capital for these hospitals is becoming an increasingly scarce resource.

- Rural communities are normally underserved by primary care physicians and enjoy very little specialist physician coverage. The community is forced to go to the larger urban centers because of the lack of accessibility to physicians in their own community.

- The quality of health care in these communities, rightly or wrongly, is usually perceived as being poor. Physicians who are perceived as excellent are usually not accepting new patients.

- Local providers respond poorly to local employer needs, although these represent an important potential source of younger insured patients.

Increasingly, physicians practicing in rural communities are finding themselves sharing with their peers the following problems:

- Managing a medical practice is becoming more difficult and taking too much time away from the practice of medicine. Rural physicians face increasing operating costs, requirements for submitting claims for payment are becoming more complex, employees are more difficult to find and retain, and contracting with payers has become a critical but confusing element of a physician practice.
- Intuitively physicians recognize that the days of the solo practitioner are numbered. However, most physicians find it difficult, if not impossible, to organize themselves for a number of reasons, one of which is the professional politics of the medical community.
- Physicians have observed the intrusion into their market by large urban medical centers, through the establishment of competing medical services or by placing competing physicians in their market. This development, coupled with the fear of encroaching managed care controlled by the larger medical centers, has made them very nervous about protecting their income and caused them to look for alternatives.
- In many cases, the physicians have already been approached by larger medical centers with offers to acquire their medical practice, in the process converting the physician into an employee. Again, intuitively, unless they are looking to retire, physicians are distrustful of this option; they do not like losing their independence.

PriCare's Approach

Convinced that the control of the local health care system in these communities should be in the hands of the medical staff, and recognizing that in virtually all cases the medical staff is too badly fragmented and too poorly organized to leverage this control effectively, PriCare created an entirely new health care delivery model to enable physicians in these smaller communities to accomplish their own personal and professional goals within an organization that was profitable in the current competitive environment.

PriCare's approach can best be explained by the example set by a leading company in the retail industry. Quite literally, every one of the kinds of rural communities traditionally underserved by the health care industry has a Wal-Mart store. This retail giant was one of the few companies that early on recognized the amount of potential business in rural America where one rarely finds K-Mart, Penney, or Sears. In essence, Wal-Mart succeeded by consolidating retailing in the rural market. Under one roof, shoppers can find a large stock of an extremely wide variety of quality products at discounted prices supported by friendly service and a physically attractive facility. Each Wal-Mart store houses a garden shop, clothing store, hardware, sporting goods, drugstore, electronics, appliances, furniture, and more. Wal-Mart has been extraordinarily successful, evidenced by full parking lots. It has reversed the out-migration of shoppers to urban areas by offering variety, quality, and competitive prices right near home. One important aspect of Wal-Mart's success is the domination of these smaller markets. In this age of encroaching managed care, it is even more important that PriCare's physician practice become the dominant player in its market.

The PriCare strategy is the health care equivalent of the Wal-Mart strategy. Its typical target market is in the southeastern states, which are generally dominated by small communities. In fact, PriCare has identified over seven hundred potential markets in just an eight-state area. The ideal market area, usually covering a county, contains a population of twenty-five to thirty-five thousand. The county seat may have two thousand to ten thousand people and typically has a small hospital with some physician presence. Ideally, the market is within twenty to fifty miles of a larger city, which has at least one major medical center. It is important that the market have an established medical presence. PriCare is not in the business of establishing health care from scratch in medically underserved areas.

PriCare moves into a new rural market by first identifying at least two top-quality primary care physicians already practicing successfully in that market. If there are not at least two physicians who fit this description, PriCare will not attempt to enter that market. More often than not, these physicians are in solo practices, and PriCare offers to acquire the non–real estate assets of each separate practice. As part of the transaction, PriCare assists the physicians in forming a new consolidated group practice; at the closing, the two previously solo practitioners become partners in their own group practice organization. PriCare manages the new group practice under a thirty-year management agreement. In essence, PriCare becomes the partner, not the employer, of these physicians. The physicians maintain both the independence and control of all medical matters, while PriCare manages the business aspects of the practice and is a source of the capital and the business expertise needed for the practice to grow.

The most important aspect of this arrangement is the fact that *the physician is not an employee*. In PriCare's judgment, this is the key to a successful physician practice management model. There are abundant unhappy examples of hospitals, both for-profit and not-for-profit, that bought physician practices, with unpleasant results. The traditional hospital model is to acquire and employ the physician with generous guaranteed salary packages. The physician soon learns that he or she makes the same amount of money whether he or she is playing golf or seeing patients, and inevitably his or her productivity declines, sometimes dramatically. The end result is an unmotivated and unhappy physician and a practice owner who ends up with much less than it thought it bought. PriCare's physician compensation model is based solely on productivity and offers physicians the ability to increase their own income by significantly participating in the upside provided through practice income growth.

After the acquisition is completed, PriCare owns the practice assets, furniture, equipment, accounts receivable, and so forth, and the former employees of the physician become PriCare employees. Under the terms of a management agreement, PriCare is reimbursed for all practice expenses from the revenues generated by the practice and receives a management fee based on a percentage of net revenues. In addition, PriCare shares with the physicians in the improvements to the consolidated practice net income compared to the prior solo practice incomes. This aspect of the relationship couples the incentives of PriCare and the practice physicians. A bad or a good decision for one party is the same for both.

Together with the physician partners, PriCare immediately begins to implement the company's own medical practice business model, which is critical if the physicians are to be positioned to control their local market. The first step is to provide a modern facility that will accommodate the newly consolidated combined practices and collateral aspects of the PriCare model. This can be accomplished either by building a new facility or by expanding one of the existing facilities, but in either case, it is the physicians, not PriCare, who will own the facility.

PriCare's business model includes the following changes to the practice:

- As soon as possible, all physicians are consolidated into one facility. In the meantime, PriCare manages each practice individually and makes improvements where indicated.

- PriCare recruits or acquires new primary care physicians as soon as possible. This is important to solve the accessibility problem, expand services, increase market share, and reverse patient out-migration.

- PriCare's model includes conversion of the consolidated practice to the PriCare Way. The new practice may be converted to the Medical Manager Computer System that is used companywide. This provides the accounting and information systems required to manage the practice in today's more demanding business environment. Additionally, PriCare's uniform business office practices and personnel policies and procedures are implemented in each new practice.
- The PriCare management team examines the feasibility of creating the consolidated practice, acquires the equipment, and initiates new ancillary services. With the increase in the number of physicians, the necessary critical mass of patients is secured to support lab, X-ray, CT scanner, ultrasound, and other equipment.
- Consolidation of referrals from the group's primary care physicians to selected high-quality physicians in each specialty creates a critical mass of patients, justifying specialists' holding office hours in the PriCare facility. In essence, PriCare brings the specialist to the patient instead of the patient's having to travel to a larger city to see the specialist. This feature of PriCare's model is extremely important. In most cases, obstetrics and gynecology specialty services are not available locally, and this one health care area alone results in much of the patient out-migration. Most younger women want to see a specialist for their delivery or for gynecological problems. Inevitably, if they leave the community, they will also direct other family members to the urban physicians for their health care needs. Reversing the trend in this single area can have a substantial positive impact, so it is usually the first specialty area in which PriCare concentrates.

- Extended hours are initiated. PriCare facilities are typically open from 8:00 A.M. to 8:00 P.M., seven days a week. These extended hours significantly increase the all-important availability and accessibility for patients.
- Urgent care services are initiated. Minor injuries can be handled by the practice on an extended-hour basis, and the ability to handle unscheduled patients during normal hours is enhanced.

PriCare places considerable emphasis on its industrial medicine program. Most smaller communities have one or more large employers, but because they are spread out, they are not always evident. A good example is Pulaski, Tennessee, a community of 7,985 people, but with sixty-five employers employing one hundred or more employees. This level of industry is not apparent from a drive through the town. These employees are an insured, mobile population who very likely travel to the nearest urban community for health care. PriCare's industrial medicine program is designed to provide preemployment services, on-the-job injury services, and physical therapy in a cost-effective and efficient manner. The number one complaint by industry is not necessarily the cost of care, but the lost productivity experienced while their employees are receiving care. PriCare's "one-stop shopping" is exactly what the employer is seeking. However, the more important role of the industrial medicine program is to gain access to an insured population that can be converted to permanent patients for the company's physician practices.

In short, as in the case of Wal-Mart, patients have access to one-stop shopping for their health care needs. Under one roof they can receive quality services that include primary care physician treatment, the latest diagnostic examinations, and, if needed, specialist care. In effect, they can receive practically any service short of inpatient hospital care or subspecialty physician services right in their own home town.

The benefits to the patients and community are improved health care services. As for the physicians, they too have numerous benefits:

- *Independence*. Physicians continue to have complete control of all medical matters and have significant participation in all other decision making.
- *Relief from the rigors of day-to-day practice management tasks*. PriCare's experience is that this is frequently the number one motivation causing physicians to examine their practice change options.
- *Access to capital for expansion of services*. Rural market physicians typically do not have the resources required to recruit new physicians or acquire the equipment necessary to provide new diagnostic ancillary services.
- *Access to a management team that has expertise in virtually all areas of practice management*. Each practice has an on-site practice administrator who reports to a corporate vice president of operations. That individual is responsible for ensuring that PriCare's practice model is implemented and that necessary corporate resources are available to the practice.
- *Increased income*. While other health care initiatives are trying to generate profits in part by reducing physician income, PriCare practice model physicians can look forward to increased income as the new and superior services they offer expand their control over their local market.

This model provides one additional enormous benefit to the physician practice. By securing the top-quality physicians in the market, being in the position to control the cost of ancillary services, and becoming in essence the gatekeeper for local industry,

PriCare's practice model effectively becomes the physician practice model of choice in the local market for managed care. In addition, the practice's success and strength in its local market make it far more difficult for other organizations, such as urban medical centers and national managed care model plans, to penetrate and fragment the local market.

Most important, patients benefit from improved quality of care. Improved accessibility to physicians and diagnostic tools is in itself an improvement, but perhaps the greatest impact comes from increased control over the treatment of the patient. A frequent complaint of rural primary care physicians is that once a patient is referred to a specialist, or referred out for a diagnostic test, the patient often does not follow through and the primary care physician is either powerless to do anything or is unaware of the lack of follow-through. By having the diagnostic tools and the specialist in-house, continuity, speed of diagnosis, and the ability of the primary care physician to consult directly with the specialist are dramatically improved. In short, appropriate treatment of the patient is more readily assured and completed on a more timely basis.

4

Agile Organizations and Health Care Collaboration

Michael H. Annison

Throughout the mature phase of industrial society, organizational boundaries were clear, the terms of competition were explicit, and market expectations were relatively predictable. Organizations concentrated on doing more of what they were already doing: carmakers made cars and grocery stores sold food. This stability provided a rationale for specialization and for evaluating the performance of individual employees, individual departments, and individual divisions within large organizations. For over one hundred years, this approach worked well. It no longer does: not in manufacturing, not in design or marketing, not in professional services, and not in health care. As Ben Owens, the chief executive at St. Bernards Regional Medical Center in Jonesboro, Arkansas, observed in an interview (personal communication, Nov. 17, 1977), "Today there are no more rules."

In the last third of the twentieth century, changes in the social, economic, and political structure of the United States have fundamentally altered how people work and how they manage the organization of work. The result of these changes is that organizations have had to become more agile to survive; doing more of what a company has always done has become, as often as not, a prescription for disaster. The explosive growth of the information society and of global telecommunications, together with the collapse of their costs, have led to a blurring of boundaries in what used to be distinct fields. Thanks to car loans, leasing schemes, car rental subsidiaries, and extended warranty insurance programs, General Motors, Ford, and Chrysler are now among the country's leading financial institutions. Grocery stores still sell food, but many also now house banking services and post office substations, prepare food, sell airline tickets, provide shoe repairs, rent videos, process film, and sell telephones.

To prosper in a rapidly changing and increasingly competitive environment, health care organizations, like all other commercial enterprises, will have to become agile, and one hallmark of their agility will be the ability to develop and manage collaborative relationships.

The Range of Collaborative Efforts

Independence was the hallmark of the industrial society; today, independence has become an expensive indulgence. Collaboration has become a competitive necessity both within and between organizations and even across traditional industry boundaries.

Collaboration Within Organizations

Agile organizations encourage collaboration among previously independent departments. In the automotive industry, Ford Motor Company adopted a collaborative approach to the design of the Ford Taurus. The Taurus was designed by employee teams made up of members from marketing, design, manufacturing, purchasing, and planning who worked together to design one of the most successful cars ever produced. Chrysler's resurgence in the 1990s has been largely the result of implementing a platform team approach—extending membership to key suppliers—to the creation of the Dodge Intrepid family of sedans, the Neon, and the redesign of the Jeep Cherokee. In the process, Chrysler cut the time and the cost of bringing these cars to market almost in half.

In financial services, Scott Jones, the chief executive of Community Bankshares in Minneapolis, Minnesota, and incoming 1999 chairman of the American Banking Association, focused on the importance of collaboration when he said: "Teamwork—every time we find success in this organization, it ultimately boils down to that important ingredient" (personal communication, June 16, 1987).

In the aircraft industry, Boeing adopted the same idea in designing and building the Boeing 777 airliner, using an approach called concurrent engineering. Like Chrysler, Boeing adopted Catia computer-based design software as the standard for its cross-functional design teams extending over Boeing's far-flung divisions, major suppliers around the world, and key customers. Because of this degree of collaboration, the 777—the first aircraft designed entirely on computer and manufactured directly from computer-generated drawings with no models, mockups, or prototypes—moved into service faster and cheaper than had been thought possible. From concept to delivery, this certified-to-fly aircraft, an extraordinarily complex machine with some three million parts, took only five years. By comparison, before collaborative cross-functional teams were introduced, it took GM, Ford, and Chrysler five to seven years to bring to market a new car, which only has some twenty-five thousand parts.

Collaboration enables organizations to respond more effectively to changing markets and changing customer expectations because collaborative teams have attributes not found in top-down organizations. First, they make it possible to move information more effectively than traditional hierarchies. Rather than communicating up, down, and across traditional organizational boundaries, agile organizations use collaborative teams to disperse information to people who need it. Second, collaborative efforts bring relevant points of view to bear on issues simultaneously rather than sequentially (thus, concurrent operations). As a result, teams are able to solve problems more quickly and at lower total cost because they share comprehensive information directly rather than dealing with partial information secondhand.

Emerging agile health care organizations have focused on fostering collaboration in three internal areas.

Improving Quality

The first area of collaboration is medical care itself, where the challenge is to improve the quality of care that doctors and hospitals provide while simultaneously lowering the costs of providing that care. Work in this area has focused on two issues: the improvement of care during a patient's hospital stay and the management of an episode of care both before and after a hospital stay itself. Doctors who used to pride themselves on their independence are finding that working with colleagues and hospital staff to develop practice guidelines and protocols can help them improve the care they provide their patients.

These guidelines, when used appropriately, provide a framework for the doctor's practice of medicine rather than a substitute for his or her professional judgment. Medical staffs and the health care systems with which they are associated are learning that collaboration can help them improve the care they provide. Collaboration is equally important in managing the care a patient receives prior to and after a hospital stay. Care coordinators work with the patient, the family, and the physician to ensure that the entire process goes smoothly. The ability to plan the patient's care prior to and after hospitalization has significant medical benefits and makes the process easier for the patient and the family.

Improving Operations

The second collaborative focus is hospital operations. Symptomatic of emerging organizational agility, physicians and hospital staff members are working together to redesign hospital clinical procedures in areas such as laboratory testing and diagnostic procedures, as well as in support areas such as dietary services. It has long been known, for example, that patients admitted to the American hospital early in the week have shorter lengths of stay than do patients who are admitted on Thursday or Friday. The reason is simple: hospital diagnostic departments and departments in other service areas have traditionally shut down over the weekend.

Structuring physician and staff schedules so that diagnostic capabilities are available on weekends makes it possible to provide consistent care for patients and decrease lengths of stay. The result is better care at lower cost. Similarly, doctors and hospitals have learned that collaboration is essential to the improvement of emergency services. The objective is emergency procedures designed to ensure that the patient understands that care begins with the first contact with a clinical person (whether it is a nurse or a doctor), that procedures are clearly explained so patients know what will happen to them during their care, and that nurses understand the importance of caring for the patient *and* their families. The result of collaborative efforts in emergency room procedures has been better care and more satisfied patients.

Developing Policy

The third area of collaboration in agile health care systems is strategic planning and the development of policy for the overall organization. Successful organizations use mechanisms such as annual planning retreats, mini-retreats focused on discussions of single issues, and joint attendance at local and national conferences by board members, doctors, and managers who attend these sessions as teams. These types of collaborative efforts are essential because the roles of board members, executives, and doctors have changed.

Board members who used to be responsible only for hospital operations have learned that they need to be much more knowledgeable about medical care and procedures. Similarly, doctors who used to focus exclusively on the practice of medicine have learned that they need to become knowledgeable about hospital operations, the financing of medicine, and issues such as community health and the development of managed care. These collaborative efforts are effective when physicians provide a clinical perspective on issues being discussed rather than representing the medical staff. At the Memorial Hermann Healthcare System (MHHS) in Houston, for example, board members, medical staff leaders, and senior managers participate in a joint annual retreat. In addition, in the course of the year, there are three or four mini-retreats, each focused on a single issue, such as managed care contracting or care for the poor. MHHS managers, physicians, and board members routinely attend conferences such as the Estes Park Institute together. The result is the creation of shared perceptions of changes in health care and a common understanding of the issues that these individuals together need to address if MHHS is to succeed in its health care mission.

Throughout the early part of this century, the metaphor for the American hospital was a three-legged stool. The belief was that strong hospitals were the result of a strong medical staff, effective board members, and strong management, each independently carrying out their individual responsibilities. The metaphor for the hospital in the 1990s is three overlapping circles: board members, medical staff leaders, and managers working together to respond to changing patient expectations, changing community needs, and the need to provide higher-quality care at lower cost.

Collaboration Across Organizations

Agile organizations recognize the importance of collaboration across traditional boundaries. Publishing companies, for example, now collaborate on the management of inventory and distribution centers and in financial services. Visa and MasterCard collaborate on issues such as fraud, abuse, and the development of automatic teller machines (ATMs).

In health care, cross-organizational collaborative efforts have taken two forms. First, hospitals have developed national cooperatives. These national cooperatives, such as the Voluntary Hospitals of America (VHA) and Premier, have enabled their members jointly to negotiate deals with national suppliers more effectively than they ever could acting independently. Participating members are able to lower costs associated with both the purchasing and inventory management of medical supplies they all routinely use. These cooperatives have also focused on the development and use of information and data systems that provide members with comparative data on the effectiveness of their individual operations. Sharing information across traditionally independent health care organizations enables members to identify opportunities for improving operations.

The second approach has focused on collaborative relationships in individual local communities. As hospitals have looked at wellness and community health, they have found that collaboration with other social service providers is essential to meeting the needs of people they serve. The Lancaster Health Alliance in Lancaster, Pennsylvania, for example, works with thirty-four community organizations, including the American Cancer Society, the Child Abuse Prevention Committee, Head Start of Lancaster, the Bureau of Police, the Urban League, the Spanish American Civic Association, and the United Way of Lancaster. The purpose of each of these relationships is to focus on the health care needs of specific populations and pool the expertise of the hospital and the collaborating organization. The result is improved access to health care and better services than any individual organization could provide by itself.

Collaboration Across Sectors

Similarly, there are growing numbers of collaborative efforts across traditionally independent sectors. In economic development, successful communities used to be the result of independent businesses' pursuing their individual interests. Now communities have found that bringing businesspeople, educators, health care providers, and public officials together is essential if they are to be successful in developing or attracting business to their community. One of the groundbreaking examples is the Research Triangle in Raleigh-Durham, North Carolina, developed in the 1960s and 1970s.

James Hunt, the state's governor, saw the public responsibility as cutting the red tape to help community leaders accomplish what needed to be done to improve economic development. Hunt was committed to collaboration and the state's working closely with private sector and not-for-profit community organizations. Community leaders had the responsibility to identify and attract business to the Raleigh-Durham area. Social service providers such as school superintendents and hospital executives were essential participants in the process because companies expected their employees and their families to have access to high-quality schools and hospitals. This same approach to collaborative economic development has been followed in other successful communities across the United States, from Silicon Valley in California to "Robot Alley" on the east coast of Florida.

In health care, collaborative arrangements across organizations are essential because of changing community expectations. The umbrella of health care is broadening and now includes a growing recognition that it is as important to keep people well as it is to care for them when they are ill. This focus on community health requires that hospital board members, health care executives, and physician leaders look beyond the hospital walls and develop ways to help people maintain their health. Successful community health efforts have targeted community education, the provision of care in settings outside the hospital, and the development of support groups for patients with diseases such as Alzheimer's and cancer. When they are effective, these community health efforts have involved hospitals, school systems, churches, businesses, community organizations, and local governments. In Jonesboro, Arkansas, for example, the St. Bernards Regional Medical Center works with state government to promote the Kids First program, which provides immunizations to young children. As a result of collaborative efforts by state government, physicians, and hospital staff, over 90 percent of the children in Craighead County and the surrounding area have had immunization shots.

The need to be able to respond effectively and efficiently to changing patient expectations and changing community needs is driving both of these types of collaborative efforts: among individuals within a single organization and among organizations with convergent health care agendas in different sectors of society. As the emphasis on wellness and community health continues to grow, these efforts and others like them will be increasingly important.

What Collaborative Arrangements Do

Agile organizations value collaborative arrangements because they enable them to gain a richer understanding of changes that will affect how they care for patients and adjust to changing community needs. They also enable organizations to accomplish what they need to do more effectively than they could operating independently.

Learning

Collaborative arrangements are important learning mechanisms for board members, physicians, and hospital staff, providing opportunities to gain richer insights into the issues that each group must deal with every day. Effective organizations learn from organizations in other fields, peer organizations in health care, and related organizations such as suppliers.

The Executive Committee (TEC) in Milwaukee, Wisconsin, is an example of one approach to learning across traditional industry boundaries. After retiring as the chief executive of his own business, Robert Norris founded TEC because he felt chief executives needed a forum to share ideas with peers. Each TEC group has approximately twelve members who meet monthly to share ideas and experiences in areas such as marketing, sales, human resources, general management, and planning. Each CEO comes from a different noncompeting industry. The benefit to health care executives who participate is significant because TEC provides an opportunity for them to understand how peers in other fields manage the same kinds of issues that they deal with every day.

Similar mechanisms exist in many communities that have established leadership programs for executives to learn more about community needs and other community organizations. These programs focus on issues such as education, health care, economic development, housing, and transportation. In Red Wing, Minnesota, the communitywide town planning project, Red Wing 2000, provides the opportunity for health care executives and other community leaders to address issues that affect community health and the well-being of the entire community.

Health care organizations such as the Estes Park Institute (EPI) provide a different and equally important opportunity for learning. Estes Park sponsors regular forums that provide an opportunity for board members, medical staff leaders, and health care executives to explore issues that affect the future of their own communities. For over thirty years, the Estes Park Institute has convened forums that address issues related to public policy, the future of health care, alternative medicine, and healthy communities. The forums are effective because they provide the opportunity for health care leaders to learn from each other and from colleagues in other organizations in other parts of the country.

Agile organizations learn from other industries and from each other. They also learn from their own suppliers in areas such as information systems and facilities management. Agile health care systems have moved beyond traditional customer-vendor relationships and formed partnerships with suppliers. These partnerships enable the suppliers and their health system clients to develop more effective products and services than they could by working independently.

On a national level, Healthcare Research and Development Institute (HRDI) serves as a forum for national health care leaders to work with leading industry suppliers. Individual HRDI working groups study issues such as the design and construction of health care facilities, hospital equipment, facilities management, and operating issues such as inventory management. Agile health care systems have individually formed partnerships with information service providers such as IBM, HBOC, and Shared Medical Systems. When they are effective, these become collaborative partnerships that enable the client system and its supplier information company to work together to meet the present and future needs of physicians and hospital staff. Similarly, agile health care systems have found it more effective to develop partnerships to manage hospital services such as food service and maintenance. Collaborative relationships with companies such as ServiceMaster and Marriott enabled them to provide high-quality services by drawing on expertise in specific areas so they can accomplish their overall purposes more effectively than they could by themselves.

The purpose of these learning relationships, whether they are within or across traditional boundaries, is to enable board members, health care executives, and physicians to avoid becoming so preoccupied with their own operations and the way they have always done things that they lose sight of opportunities to continue to improve patient care and meet the needs of the communities they serve. As health care continues to change, these relationships will be increasingly important learning mechanisms, enhancing and extending traditional mechanisms.

Accomplishing Work

A second function of collaborative relationships is to enable participants to accomplish work more effectively than they could operating independently. The catchphrase for agile organizations may very well be: "I may have to do it myself, but that doesn't mean I have to do it alone."

Agile organizations have developed joint ventures, strategic alliances, corporate agreements, contract arrangements, and other mechanisms that enable them to work effectively with other providers or vendors to meet the needs of patients and communities. In Houston, the Memorial Hermann Healthcare System and the Sisters of Charity developed a joint venture for expanding outpatient clinical services and developing insurance products. Memorial and the Sisters of Charity shared the goal of moving services beyond traditional hospital walls. They also believed that health care organizations could effectively develop managed care products and, most important, they believed they could accomplish these goals more effectively by working together than they could by pursuing them independently. The result was the development of a strategic alliance formed to expand clinical services and provide competitive managed care products to individuals and organizations.

Some strategic alliances cross traditional industry boundaries. Over the past decade, numerous Blue Cross–Blue Shield organizations have dealt with changes in health care by converting to publicly traded companies or merging to form larger organizations. In Arkansas, Blue Cross chose a different strategy: it developed strategic alliances with leading community hospitals across the state. The purpose of the alliances is to enable Blue Cross and its partners to improve the management of medical care, develop interactive information systems that move the right information to the right person at the right time, and manage risk collaboratively. To accomplish these goals, Blue Cross decentralized its clinical and marketing functions by establishing regional offices that have enabled it and its partners more effectively to coordinate marketing plans, share clinical information, and improve services to patients and doctors with whom they work.

The point of these alliances, whether they are reflected in national organizations such as Voluntary Hospitals of America, cross-industry groups such as HRDI, or alliances in individual communities such as Lancaster and Houston, is to position health care systems to respond to a changing environment more effectively than they could if they were acting independently. These efforts have three benefits. First, agile organizations learn and respond more effectively to changes in health care. Second, participating organizations develop new capabilities and services more effectively than they could by themselves, and third, they reduce the risks associated with change by drawing on the insights, skills, and expertise of collaborating organizations with different capabilities.

Collaboration and Competition

As they have developed collaborative relationships, health care organizations have had to grapple with learning how to manage relationships that are, as often as not, simultaneously collaborative and competitive. Although the phenomenon is still relatively new in health care, companies in fields such as financial services, the computer industry, and the automotive business have found ways to do this. In financial services, banks compete and simultaneously collaborate in credit operations such as Visa. In the automotive industry, car dealers co-locate in specific areas of communities, realizing that the goal of increasing the potential pool of buyers by attracting the maximum number of people shopping for cars to one part of town by cooperating with rival dealers is not incompatible with the goal of competing with those same dealers' sales. In many communities, antique dealers have adopted the same approach, as have jewelers.

In health care, these types of collaborative-and-competitive relationships occur in three areas. The first is in the relationship between doctors and hospitals and among doctors themselves: the question is which services will be provided in which locations.

As they develop, all technologies get smaller, faster, and cheaper. Notebook computers, for example, can have more power and more capabilities than mainframe computers had twenty years ago. In health care, this pattern means that as they develop, medical technologies migrate from the nation's teaching and research centers to tertiary hospitals, primary and secondary centers, doctors' offices, and in some cases other community locations and even the home. X-ray machines have moved from the hospital to the doctor's office, and magnetic resonance imaging has moved from tertiary hospitals to community hospitals across the country.

This pattern of technological innovation means that hospitals and members of their medical staff compete for who will provide which services, while simultaneously collaborating on how to improve care for patients in the hospital. At the same time, technological innovation has led to an erosion of boundaries among doctors themselves. Specialists who used to practice in distinct fields now find themselves competing with the hospital as well as with colleagues who have access to new medical technologies and can provide a wider range of services for patients. Radiologists, for example, now compete with cardiologists over who will interpret diagnostic procedures, and specialist surgeons compete with each other over who will have privileges to do which kinds of procedures.

At the same time, hospitals and other health care providers compete over who will provide which kinds of services. The boundaries between general community hospitals, long-term care providers, and specialty hospitals used to be clear, just as they were clear between hospitals and providers such as hospice and home health care agencies. Now, changes in patient and community expectations, as well as changes in public policy and reimbursement mechanisms, have compelled previously independent organizations to rethink which services they provide and how they will provide them. Specialty hospital companies such as Health South, for example, have developed relationships with general community hospitals while they simultaneously expand into the general hospital business itself. Community organizations such as the Visiting Nurses Association (VNA) have developed collaborative relationships with hospitals, many of which are competitors, as the hospital and the VNA seek to meet a growing demand for home health care services.

On an even broader level, there are collaboration and competition among health systems and insurance companies as each has diversified into fields outside its traditional industry boundaries. Health systems such as Memorial Hermann have developed insurance products, and insurance companies such as Anthem (formerly Blue Cross of Indiana) have acquired medical practices and begun to provide direct care to patients. In each case, the health system and the insurance company have had to find ways to work together, knowing that they are working collaboratively while at the same time competing with one another and collaborating with other health care and insurance organizations.

These patterns, well developed and more generally accepted in other fields, are still relatively new in health care, and relationships are still awkward and in many cases contentious. Agile organizations have been successful because they have been willing to embrace rather than resist these types of relationships and because they have been able to develop mechanisms to manage them effectively.

Managing New Relationships

Where they have managed these collaborative relationships effectively, agile organizations have focused on four issues. The first is on strategy and values rather than structures and operations. The inherited focus on operations highlights existing organizational arrangements and bureaucratic concerns rather than values and the strategic opportunities enabled by relationships. Under these conditions, collaboration is difficult, if not impossible. Collaborative efforts are effective when leaders focus on values and strategy, knowing that operations will have to change to take advantage of new opportunities.

Second, collaborative efforts are effective when partners look at the long-term benefits of relationships rather than their inevitable short-term start-up difficulties. Effective partners have been willing to change the way they operate rather than continuing to do things the way they have always been done or insisting that their partners adopt their own policies, systems, and procedures. One of the first tasks following the 1997 merger of Memorial Health Care System and the Hermann Hospital System was to develop a new statement of mission, purpose, and values that drew on the strengths of the two historically strong organizations rather than insist that either conform to what the other was doing. The attention in effective collaborative relationships is on the continuing work that needs to be done to adjust to new realities and changing patient and community expectations.

Third, in effective collaborative efforts, partners scrutinize the benefits of the relationship to alleviate, minimize, or eliminate areas of low-value competition or overlapping services. When these relationships are effective, collaborating organizations focus on patients and community needs rather than on institutional tidiness. There will inevitably be overlap, duplication, and competition. Agile organizations seek to meet the needs of people they serve rather than concentrate on institutional efficiency and the difficulties inherent in any collaborative effort.

Fourth, agile organizations share information and are willing to deal with difficult issues. Partners tell each other everything rather than hold back or operate with hidden agendas. In effective relationships, partners share their hopes, perceptions, and pragmatic information, which enables them to deal effectively with the inevitable challenges they face.

Changes in the social, economic, and political structure of the United States and the impact of those changes in health care mean that, as Ben Owens observed, "there are no more rules." Successful health care organizations now and in the future will be agile and able to respond to changes in patient expectations, community needs, and public policy. We will see additional changes in the future as hospital and physician groups continue to change in response to clinical and financial pressures they face, as complementary medicine continues to grow, and as organizations focus increasingly on community health. It is clear that the future will be very different from the present and that organizations that cling to what worked in the past will have grave difficulty succeeding in that very different future.

5

Leading the Agile Health Care Enterprise

Roderick Gilkey, Gary R. Lieberman

Maintaining the status quo is not an option for the increasingly competitive, cost-sensitive health care industry. Leaders face the alternative of changing faster than the environment or falling behind. The search for new solutions and new leadership models is a critical part of every executive's job. There is a paradoxical effect associated with developing new approaches to managing, because new organizational models that are designed to provide new solutions also create unanticipated consequences and unexpected dilemmas. It is a fact of organizational life that today's problems were yesterday's solutions. The agile organization, as a new management model, is no exception. It is an innovative approach that has the potential to configure human and capital resources to achieve unprecedented levels of service quality, speed of response, and customer satisfaction—outcomes that are vital to the survival and growth of health care systems.

The challenge of developing the leadership capacity for agile organizations is formidable. Who will lead these agile organizations? From where will these leaders emerge? Will they simply emerge in response to the new challenges, or will we need to prepare them? Before such issues can be meaningfully addressed, we need to be very clear about the kind of leadership required to create and sustain the agile enterprise.

Describing the definitive leadership requirements of agile organizations may be as daunting a task as looking for any type of definitive certainty. The challenge may be analogous to Kierkegaard's likening the search for the truth to looking in a dark room for a black cat that is not there. At this early stage, we can identify the leadership competencies required to lead an agile organization only by successive approximation. We cannot fully identify these leaders; we must discover them. This chapter provides a preliminary discussion of the challenges associated with leadership of the agile enterprise. It is based on observations and experiences with leaders of health care and other organizations that are already achieving higher levels of agility and performance in response to new industry challenges.

There are five defining features of leaders within agile organizations that profoundly affect the leadership requirements of the future:

- *Personality:* possessing the optimal blend of cognitive and emotional competencies
- *Strategic clarity:* knowing what business you are in
- *Collaboration capacity:* understanding how to form internal and external alliances to achieve strategic results
- *Customer focus:* sensing the shifting needs and priorities of key constituencies
- *Anticipatory learning:* understanding how to gain knowledge in advance of the need to apply it, and making changes before they are required

None of these interrelated competencies is new. What is new is the particular combination of skill sets required and the extent to which these capacities must become fully deployed to achieve the levels of organizational performance necessary to succeed in the changing health care environment. This calls for new kinds of leadership provided by leaders with personality types, skills, backgrounds, and aspirations that differ from those of their predecessors. These differences are the subject of this chapter.

Personality Dimensions of the Agile Leader

In his classic work, *The Lonely Crowd: A Study of the Changing American Character* (1950), sociologist David Riesman described three archetypal personality styles: the tradition directed, the inner directed, and the other directed. The tradition-directed personality provides valuable stabilizing influence during times of continuity but a less reliable path forward in times of rapid change. In an environment of unpredictable change, applying lessons from the past is often maladaptive. For individuals and organizations living in an environment of discontinuous change, the past is not prologue to the future. Applying traditional formulas easily produces dysfunctional outcomes. In competitive arenas, repeating past practices to ensure future success often guarantees failure.

The inner-directed character achieves focus and direction from his or her internal ideals and aspirations. A strong inner vision and a relentless determination to overcome all obstacles between themselves and their goals drive these individuals. Their aspirations and achievement may have little to do with the needs or ambitions of others. At the extreme, such a character can be described as a self-made man who worships his creator. Mercifully, those who achieve great influence and wealth often turn to more philanthropic and community-oriented activities later in life. Riesman cites a number of America's early capitalists such as Rockefeller, Carnegie, and, later, Henry Ford as prime examples.

From today's health care industry, Len Abramson exhibits some of these inner-directed characteristics. Abramson was a pharmacist and an entrepreneur who built U.S. Healthcare Inc. into a multi-billion-dollar managed care organization that Aetna later purchased for a little over $8 billion. Recently he pledged a $100 million gift from the Abramson Family Foundation, a trust fund he and his wife established and direct in support of numerous causes, for the creation of the Leonard and Madlyn Abramson Family Cancer Research Institute at the University of Pennsylvania Cancer Center.

Riesman was particularly interested in the other-directed style, a Willie Lomanesque character tending to lack the clarity of self-definition and constancy of purpose necessary to act autonomously and authentically. Profoundly alienated from the roots of tradition or the stabilizing influence of identity, such individuals respond primarily to the external prompting of others. In psychological terms such personalities are variously described as displaying "field dependence," "codependence," or an "external locus of control."

In the corporate environment, these other-directed individuals have been satirized over the years in popular productions such as *How to Succeed in Business Without Really Trying* and, more recently, *Wall Street*. The other-directed personality is at best a shrewd opportunist, at worst a driven manipulator. This other-directed personality is of particular interest in the present context, because the core competences of this type of individual could be described as agility and fluidity. Responding as they do to the dictates of external influences, they become extraordinarily adept at responding to the moment.

At first glance, it might seem that such a style, which is based on its capacity to be attuned and responsive to external stimuli, might be ideal characteristics for leaders of an agile organization. However, on closer examination, the limitations and liabilities of such a character style become apparent. The other-directed character's lack of capacity to develop deep commitments to enduring values, guiding principles, or elevating aspirations creates organizations that are focused on short-term, tactical outcomes rather than long-term, strategic achievements. Even if these immediate tactical goals are presented as strategic objectives, such as earnings records, they fail to elicit the emotional commitment from employees necessary to achieve sustained levels of exemplary performance. It requires little psychological insight to discern that people do not get up in the morning excited to go to work because they can't wait to generate higher quarterly earnings, or because their organization has such a great business plan. Instead, people are motivated to invest in organizations that have a clear sense of purpose—one that is focused on providing goods or services that matter in some way to others.

For example, many critics of Columbia/HCA (CHCA) point to tactics that might be called other-directed as one reason for the problems the organization began suffering in 1997. While building a financially successful company, the senior leadership aggressively focused on pleasing Wall Street and forcing an expense-oriented, centralized strategy within the organization, even as they were buying new hospitals and other health-related businesses and pursuing rapid growth. Instead of taking steps to incorporate the new acquisitions into the company, recognizing the individual cultures and positions in the community, CHCA appeared more to swallow them whole, forcing them into a CHCA mold, making them accept the corporate moniker, and often angering the physicians, staff, and communities. At times, if an acquisition refused to accept changes or if the financial results did not meet planned standards, they were closed. In some cases, when terms of purchase could not be agreed on with a provider, Columbia constructed a competitive hospital to attempt to force the original target out of business. As a result, when legal problems and other concerns arose against Columbia, senior leaders had nowhere to turn for support among hospitals, staff, communities, and stockholders, and they were forced out. It is fair to say that many welcome the difficulties. The new leadership, led by new chairman and CEO Thomas Frist, Jr., is slowing down and trying to refocus the organization on ethics and quality care, while also allowing individual entities to drop the Columbia name, all while remaining cost conscious. However, regardless of future changes and the probability of future success, the company will never reach the vision set by former CEO Rick Scott, at least not in the way he envisioned it.

The essence of the agile leader is the ability to help others see how their daily work is significant, in other words, how it contributes to the changing needs of people around them. In that sense, agile leaders humanize the workplace by appealing to a sense of purpose and mobilizing the creative capacities of their fellow human beings to achieve that purpose. This is a lesson Columbia/HCA is now learning.

Drawing on Riesman's observations in thinking about leading agile organizations, we can begin to draw some conclusions about what these leaders will *not* be. They will not be chosen as successors because of a traditional portfolio of skills and successes. We should expect these new leaders to have histories that reflect both successes and setbacks in dealing with adversity and challenges. Their value to their organizations will be a function of both what they have learned from experience and what they have, in effect, unlearned. The agile leader will be at once informed by the past while unfettered by it. Knowing the relative value of past experience allows them to set aside previous lessons and practices in order to open themselves up to new learning and innovative responses. This openness or *tentativeness*, as Erik Erikson (1968, p. 156) once referred to it, is based on a healthy awareness of the limits of the lessons of experience and the liability of precedent-driven strategies. Thus, the agile leader will not develop his or her competence or confidence by replicating past successes. Instead, this person will rely on his or her ability to create environments and processes that allow the organization to engage in relentless questioning of the very precedents that created their success as an enterprise. The confidence of the agile leader is based on a respect and faith in people and the processes used to help them successfully engage their intellects in the service of the shared aspirations to which they have committed their lives.

Thus, the agile leader displays some of the competencies associated with each style. Although the agile leader is not primarily directed by tradition, it is clear that such leaders are mindful of the traditions and values of their organizations. They can promote aggressive change strategies because they are clear about what to preserve from the past: the mission, purpose, and values of the organization. This is the quality that Collins and Porras observed in the leadership of the eighteen organizations they described in *Built to Last: Successful Habits of Visionary Companies* (1994). They cited companies such as Disney, Hewlett-Packard, 3M, Johnson & Johnson, Procter & Gamble, Merck, Sony, Motorola, and Nordstrom as institutions whose leaders successfully balanced a commitment to tradition-based mission and values with an insistence on innovation to meet the challenges of the future. Their records speak for themselves: these companies outperformed the general stock market by a factor of twelve since 1925 (Collins and Porras, 1996, p. 65). In these organizations, the high degree of clarity and consensus about who they are and what they stand for allows the energy that would otherwise be expended resolving these issues to be focused instead on innovating and changing to fulfill their organization's mission better. In short, clarity about what does not change creates the opportunity to put all available resources into what does. Agile leadership clears the path to change and innovation by providing a clear voice that articulates a constancy of purpose. In so doing the capacity to innovate is legitimated and supported. This is a hallmark of agile leadership.

Johnson & Johnson's handling of the Tylenol poisonings in 1982 illustrates how agile leadership uses tradition and clarity to manage successfully under all circumstances. The Johnson & Johnson philosophy and culture are embodied in what most call "The Credo," a four-paragraph vision and mission statement put into place in the 1940s by chairman Robert Wood Johnson. The Credo outlines the company's responsibilities: first to provider and patient, to employee, to community, and to stockholder. In 1979, chairman Jim Burke challenged his organization as to whether The Credo remained important and timely. After much debate, the company employees decided the values it espoused continued to guide the company in its actions. That is why, when seven people died in 1982 by ingesting cyanide-laced Tylenol, Burke could comfortably accept responsibility on behalf of the entire organization and pull all Tylenol off store shelves, regardless of short-term cost, estimated at $100 million, and the effect on the stock. In order to keep true to the Johnson & Johnson values, this was the appropriate action. In the long term, this has been shown to be the correct decision. It takes a strong and agile leader to manage under all circumstances, and it is not always the one that companies take. Contrast Burke's actions with those of Exxon after the *Exxon Valdez* oil spill, considered by many to be an illustration of ineffective leadership and crisis management.

In addition to the focus on tradition, the agile leader exhibits features of the inner-directed style. Not content to wait for fate to determine fortune, the agile leader provides great energy and direction toward promoting change. Agility means moving with alacrity toward higher levels of achievement in the service of lofty ambitions. The agile leader is driven by inner forces, but in a manner that engages others so they are able to lead their organizations toward growth rather than establish personal empires. Finally, the agile leader displays fluidity and adaptiveness, elements of an other-directed style. He or she is responsive to environmental flux and supportive of others who must also adapt to unpredictable change.

Although we can see elements of many previously identified styles in the agile leader, including in this case elements of tradition, inner directedness, and other directedness, there is a sense in which agility as a leadership style supersedes all of them. The agile leader is none of these styles but related to all. These leaders will transcend previous typologies of the executive whether depicted in Riesman's terms or as the organization man (Whyte, 1956), the gamesman (Maccoby, 1976), or simply as a leader (Zaleznik, 1977; Kotter, 1990). All of these terms are likely to be lacking in specificity and accuracy. For example, even the most basic definition of the leader as being one who has followers is questionable in this context. Certainly leaders of agile organizations do in a sense have traditional followers, but their achievements are arguably a function of having peers, colleagues, and coworkers who serve in a network of distributive leadership that mobilizes and magnifies collective accomplishments.

The argument here is not that we need to create new kinds of leaders or different personality types for new leadership roles. The issue is one of selecting and developing new kinds of leaders from the available pool of talent. The agile leader is not a new personality type, heretofore unknown or unavailable. In fact, a look at the long tradition of literary characters from Homer to the present will identify remarkable consistencies in the types and range of personalities. What changes over time are the types of personalities selected and promoted to positions of leadership. This may be one of the most important and least understood dilemmas in leadership. By what criteria and through what processes do we define and select our leaders? Traditional formulas are of little utility in rapidly changing circumstances. Thus, the search for new types of leaders must be based on strategic, explicit, and consensual selection criteria. We are suggesting that there are specific personality characteristics required of individuals who can successfully lead agile enterprises. These competencies and characteristics are selected in concert with the organizational requirements of the agile enterprise.

Organizational Requirements of the Agile Enterprise

Strategic Clarity

Knowing what business you are in may seem like an obvious and minimal requirement for a leader. However, in an environment of turbulent and nonlinear change, this is no easy task. The business you were in yesterday may not be the business you are in tomorrow, and as important, even if it remains approximately the same, you are very unlikely to remain in that business in the same way. The near demise of British Airways (BA) provides a case in point.

When Colin Marshall took over at BA in 1993, the airline was suffering staggering financial losses, the worst in its history. It had a correspondingly low level of customer satisfaction. Indeed, BA had come to stand for "bloody awful" in the public's view. The airline's new leadership created one of the greatest turnaround stories in modern corporate history, perhaps best summarized by Marshall's interpretation of one of the key changes: "It took me eighteen months to convince people that we are not in the airline business, we are in the customer service business" (Prokesch, 1995, p. 108). The understanding that the business exists to serve people's transportation needs makes it possible to avoid the confusion of means and ends. The purpose of British Airways, in Marshall's view, was to provide the highest level of customer satisfaction in providing for their transportation. With this in view, his team initiated the campaign, "The world's favorite airline." In this context, flying airplanes is a means, not an end; satisfying the needs of the traveling public is the end.

We are sorry to say that we are not at a loss to find examples of leaders who lost their focus and failed to see what business they were in. IBM's attachment to the mainframe is perhaps the most dramatic example of this confusion. IBM is in business to foster organizational performance through the application of advanced technologies. The mainframe was one means of doing so. Unfortunately, a number of IBM's key leaders lost the ability to differentiate between means and ends, and they construed the mainframe to be a part of IBM's core identity or purpose. Had this misguided view not been unchecked, America could have lost one of its finest companies.

Although its stock value recovered from its 1980s lows, the loss of strategic focus and clarity on the part of key IBM leaders opened the door in hardware, software, consulting, and education to a number of other companies that are now major competitors in the industry. In this context, IBM's new CEO, Lou Gerstner, was probably correct when he stated early in his tenure, "The last thing IBM needs is a vision" (Morris, 1997, p. 71). What IBM needed was not a vision of the future but an understanding of the present and an appreciation of the past: who they were, how they created value, and why customers needed them. In short, IBM needed to rediscover what business it was in so it could regenerate the company and build on its great record of success. Gerstner helped force this rediscovery by realigning many of the traditional sales functions around industries such as health care and by focusing on other services, such as consulting, which went back to the original IBM purpose: providing technology solutions to foster the success of all of its customers. IBM is now back in business providing solutions to problems of customers, including health care customers.

Maintaining strategic clarity during times of transition is particularly difficult. Luckily there are examples of success. One of them is John Henry, the CEO of two Atlanta hospitals, Crawford Long and Emory University Hospital. With a view to making the new organization, Emory Hospitals, increasingly customer focused while gaining operational efficiency and strategic clarity and maintaining what made each hospital successful in the past, Henry sponsored an educational partnership with Disney University.

Disney, a company that has achieved success balancing purpose, mission, and practice, has sought to share its knowledge and experience with others, to allow leaders and managers to take the competencies exhibited within the entertainment company and adapt them to their own organizations. Bringing together over 130 hospital directors in a series of retreats, Disney staff discussed with hospital managers best demonstrated practices in achieving levels of customer satisfaction and profitability in service settings. As a result, Emory Hospitals' management was able to determine how to transfer appropriate Disney operating practices to improve every patient encounter, including parking, reception, room services, and even what Disney refers to as "the bill-paying experience." Combining a traditional hospital enterprise with the creative capacities and operating precision of Disney is a form of nontraditional leadership that will become more frequent in the most successful organizations. Staging retreats with Disney created a context for others to think outside the box and look at their particular service area with a fresh perspective. Mobilizing the capacity of employees to find new ways to leverage their internal and external resources to achieve greater effectiveness is one of the most important products of agile leadership.

Collaborative Capacity

In a classic *Harvard Business Review* article, Abraham Zaleznik (1977) provided the foundation of contemporary leadership theory when he introduced the distinction between managers and leaders. Zaleznik noted that one of the primary differences is the depth of the relationship that managers and leaders achieve with others. Managers tend to form superficial instrumental relationships with others that lack emotional depth and knowledge. In contrast, an agile leader displays the ability to form much deeper relationships based on levels of empathy and understanding virtually unknown to managers. As a result, leaders are able to understand, motivate, and inspire others, often eliciting deep emotional allegiances and profound commitments in the process. These capacities extend to people inside and outside their immediate organizations.

This ability to transcend traditional loyalties and relationships is vitally important as health care continues to evolve and consolidate and as new forms of health care delivery develop. It becomes imperative for the agile leader to bridge traditional boundaries and alliances in what is, at its root and despite its constant innovations, a highly conservative industry.

The Minnesota marketplace is one region where leaders are exhibiting a great deal of agility on all sides. Like much of the rest of the country, the cost of health care to companies' bottom lines prompted business to demand changes in the way care was delivered and paid for. Minnesota's response was to create the Buyers Health Care Action Group (BHCAG), a coalition of twenty-six large Twin Cities–based self-insured employers representing approximately 400,000 employees, retirees, and dependents in a four-state area around Minneapolis–St. Paul (Robinson, 1997, p. 61). The ability of employers to collaborate has changed greatly—and continues to change—the way health care is provided, although its overall purpose remains to offer high-quality, efficient, cost-effective care. BHCAG also stresses provider competition, increased consumer knowledge and responsibility, and better communication among all system participants.

In order to succeed under this scenario, provider organizations had to react quickly and aggressively to change the way they delivered care. They integrated and consolidated services and better organized how their organizations delivered patient care. Methods of communication, to both the employer and the community, also increased. One organization that has been successful in adapting to the new situation, and which many consider a model for the integrated delivery system, is Allina. Allina operates nineteen hospitals, seven nursing homes, and fifty-six clinics, with 12,400 physicians and 21,200 employees, across four states. In order to create Allina in 1994, two organizations, the managed health care organization Medica and HealthSpan, the fifth largest not-for-profit (in 1993) secular health care system in the United States, merged. These two organizations were themselves made up from two large health plans, a regional health care system, and a network of independent hospitals.

Allina's success at creating a hospital-based system and health plan is due in part to its agile leadership. The leaders of the merging organizations reacted quickly and strategically to the needs of its customers—in this case, BHCAG and patients. It has created a single purpose for existing: "to provide an excellent health care experience for its customers" (Tam, 1997, p. 59). This purpose has led to a vision of being the recognized innovator in improving the health of the communities Allina serves, as well as a willingness—in many ways, a recognized need—to work with its corporate, government, and community groups to meet its goals. In practice, it strives to take certain steps organized to balance the use of technology and a customer focus (Tam, 1997, p. 60):

- Work to understand the needs of the customer.
- Focus the organization on serving the customer, using technology and every human interaction.
- Commit resources and be willing to alter organizational structures and accountabilities as needed.
- Enlist input and support from every internal and external constituency with which Allina deals.
- Show consistency. Follow through on commitments.
- Maintain momentum. Reward and provide incentives appropriately to do so.

The leaders at Allina will need to maintain their agility and willingness to collaborate in order to continue their success. Within the Minnesota market and region, BHCAG became concerned because of the system consolidation that has occurred. A handful of managed care organizations and providers, including Allina, provide the majority of care in the region. As a result, the business group is experimenting with more direct contracting between employees and physician groups, bypassing the traditional payer parties. To maintain organizational success, Allina leadership will need to adapt to the new marketplace and the new contracting arrangements.

Customer Focus

The agile leader's knowledge of and focus on customers transcends attempts to understand and manage through systems of measurement and assessment. In a *60 Minutes* interview with Diane Sawyer in February 1991, Disney's CEO Michael Eisner called formal marketing research "a crock," explaining that people will respond to marketing research questionnaires based on social desirability rather than true sentiment. He relies instead on his uncanny sense of what the customers wants in his decision making. This intuitive approach is based on a more in-depth relationship with an American public he understands well. The ability to have this understanding of and relationship with customers provides a level of awareness of customer needs and expectations that prompts agile responses to achieve changing requirements. Treating customer needs with empathy and depth of commitment allows even the largest organizations to become more agile in an effort to be responsive.

Leveraging its experience managing the information needs of the 1996 and 1998 Olympics, IBM entered into a collaboration with Southwestern Bell and Kodak to create new kinds of solutions for health care providers and patients. One initiative, called Project Spectrum, provided Barnes Jewish Christian Health System (BJC) in St. Louis with a central data repository that collects data from multiple legacy systems to give caretakers easy and immediate access to clinical patient information. As the project evolves, it will link all of BJC's hospitals and its thirty-five hundred affiliated physicians to the central data repository. What is termed a "project" is in reality a new organization, consisting of thirteen hospitals, six nursing homes, and more than one hundred ambulatory care delivery sites. Through multiple creative collaborations, BJC, working with IBM and its partners, was able to convert multiple information systems—eight clinical, five laboratory, six radiology, and eight patient accounting—into one agile central system that is now meeting the needs of its multiple customer groups. This ability to create a viable virtual organization organized around, in this case, the providers of health care services for a large metropolitan population is a prime example of how agility can make a difference in achieving new levels of organizational performance. With proper leadership and strategic clarity, even the largest organizations can create increasingly high levels of customer satisfaction by responding to their needs with agility.

Regina Herzlinger, the Nancy R. McPherson Professor of Business Administration at the Harvard Business School, has studied health care delivery systems for twenty-five years and has recently written *Market Driven Health Care: Who Wins, Who Loses in the*

Transformation of America's Largest Service Industry (1997). In it, Herzlinger cites the many changes that American society is undergoing in the way we live our lives. As a result, she believes that health care must radically transform itself around the needs of its users. At present, the system is often inconvenient in terms of both location and access. Herzlinger points to the cancer treatment center, Salick Health Care, and Pearle Vision as examples of the "focused factory" concept that will provide Americans with health care that is of high quality, is cost-effective, and is convenient. She expands on the idea of patient-focused care by placing all of the segments of the health care system either under one roof or within easy reach.

Whether Herzlinger's ideas are realized fully or not, agile leaders will need to focus even more than their predecessors on meeting the needs of those who use their services. BJC has attempted to do this through Project Spectrum. Allina is working to create a culture whose focus is the customer. This was the case when Allina partnered with IBM to create the Allina Health Village, a web site accessible to patients and others that provides information about Allina and about health care issues. In addition, both have expanded the reach of their clinics and their services out into their communities, to provide better and more convenient access.

Anticipatory Learning

We have thus far characterized agile leadership as being strategically focused, collaborative, and customer oriented. None of these features would be sufficient without an insistent drive for learning as a form of competitive advantage and quality improvement. The learning process in organizations is often inhibited by traditional structures and practices that regulate the flow of information required to perceive emerging opportunities and threats. The barriers to learning and performance improvement have led to passionate calls for boundarylessness, reengineering, flattening, or delayering from numerous CEOs trying to expedite change in their organizations. Such efforts, in their more reasonable forms, are an attempt to create "healthy hierarchies" (Ashkenas, Ulrich, Jick, and Kerr, 1995), organizations with permeable boundaries that facilitate a freer flow of information and a faster acquisition of knowledge. Organizations designed to expedite learning across boundaries—be they vertical (between levels), horizontal (across functions), or external (between organizations)—share an ability to understand and respond to environmental changes more rapidly. This is the essence of what GE's CEO Jack Welch has referred to as "speed, simplicity and self-confidence" (Tichy and Charan, 1989). The combination of knowing your business, your customers, and your people in such an information-rich environment allows you to elevate your organization's performance with greater speed and precision. Welch and GE have proved this over and over. Whether through formal programs or informal processes, barriers to transmission of information and best practices are systematically removed at GE. An innovation in the accounting department can move from one sector to another so that production processes at a manufacturing site can be improved. Enhancing organizational agility by creating more permeable boundaries can occur on four critical dimensions (Ashkenas, Ulrich, Jick, and Kerr, 1995, p. 43):

- *Information* moves from information closely held or integrated at the top to open information sharing throughout the organization.
- *Competence* moves from leadership skills exercised at senior levels and technical skills exercised at lower levels to competencies distributed though all levels.
- *Authority* moves from decisions made only at the top to decisions made all along the line, at whatever points are appropriate.
- *Rewards* moves from rewards based on position to rewards and incentives based on accomplishment.

Allina's policies and procedures reflect these elements, which are part of a deliberate strategy to increase the flow of information, power, authority, and skills across its multiparty organization. As another example, Mayo Clinic Jacksonville partnered with Cerner several years ago to institute a paperless record system within the clinic. All notes and records, from check-in to bedside to check-out, are automated. The new system ultimately will make record keeping more consistent and clear, and provide better service to patients and payers. Leadership was willing to pay for the system and to train everyone, staff and physicians, in its use.

One issue with installing the system was the radical change in behavior it required, particularly on the part of physicians, who are accustomed to writing notes in whatever form they wish. Mayo's solution, as described by staff physician Prince Zachariah, was to mandate this change, linking compliance and utilization of the technology with the physicians' compensation and incentives. Zachariah, a key physician leader in the Mayo system, makes it clear that the dedicated commitment of top leaders determined to serve their customers better was a vital ingredient in this successful conversion to new technology. This insistent drive to learn, innovate, and improve continuously, and the willingness to make difficult decisions that are best for the organization and its customers, is a core attribute of the agile leader.

Finally, we have the example of our own system, Emory Health Care, whose leaders created the Learning Council, designed to improve the system's ability to learn and transmit knowledge. The council initiated a leadership competency development program that provided an instrument to help leaders assess their individual strengths and weaknesses with respect to a set of identified competencies. Such instruments are usually designed by identifying a set of competencies that have allowed current and past leaders to be effective and using those traits as a benchmark to rate developing leaders. This retrospective approach assumes that the skills required for past and current success will be equally viable in the future.

Demonstrating what we are describing as agile, future-focused leadership, John Henry, CEO of the hospitals, insisted that the competencies that were to be identified for constructing a competency model and rating instrument be defined on the basis of future leadership competencies. The task then called for anticipatory learning: dealing with future challenges by creating scenarios depicting what the system might become and what would be required of those individuals who would lead it.

Agile leaders facilitate learning processes that direct the organization's attention forward to the future. In doing so they develop the intuitive and imaginative capacities of people who can create strategies to achieve future success.

Conclusion

Advances in the practice of management carry the promise of better performance and the burden of new leadership challenges. Organizational agility is such an advance. The leaders of agile organizations must themselves be agile: committed to rapid, customer-focused responsiveness that is both flexibly innovative and predictably consistent. Leadership is ultimately an expression of character. In the case of the agile leader, that character rests on a solid bedrock of principle, an inner faith in one's vision, confidence in one's hopes for the future, and an unswerving commitment to the betterment of the institutions that serve the human community.

6

Adapting to Consumer-Driven Health Care

James R. Cramer, Wendy H. Lyons

Intensifying competition is driving the need for flexible, innovative approaches to the very definition of health care services, no less than to their delivery. The attraction of agility is that it offers a systematic framework for health care innovation that is closely coupled to market realities. Consistent with the agility model, Scottsdale Health Care (SHC) has worked cooperatively with its diverse customers to manage health care services in an integrated way rather than to improve the delivery of segmented, episodic care. One major objective was to create a communitywide health and wellness system by finding creative ways to collaborate with health care professionals and other health care and community organizations. Thus, in place of a long-term strategic plan that would limit its flexibility and its ability to respond to evolving community needs, SHC identified near-term (an eighteen-month horizon) business drivers that determine how it needs to deal with changes in the local and national marketplace:

- Managing risk, which encompasses efforts to review continually and participate in a variety of payment mechanisms and methodologies
- Cost initiatives, which focus on opportunities to improve processes, increasing efficiency, outcome, and satisfaction

- Constituents served, which provide mechanisms to project and increase market share through innovative programming and delivery designs that reflect constant vigilance to consumer needs and wants
- Primary care, which refers to initiatives that address the growing needs of customers for this service

Through SHC-owned physician practices and the primary care physicians on its medical staffs, SHC was able to increase access to service through participation in a multitude of health plans with wide geographic coverage.

In response to these drivers, which emerged in the late 1980s and early 1990s, health care organizations have significantly increased their expenditures, and their dependence, on information technology. One goal was to adapt to the economics of managed care by automating business processes and using information to reduce high-cost acute care, without sacrificing quality, and by relocating care to ambulatory settings: the office, the clinic, or the home.

Today, even as health care organizations continue to be pressured by managed care, they face another new market force: informed and assertive health care consumers who demand that each health care organization be capable of responding to their unique expectations and to those of an entire population of like-minded people. These consumers have little tolerance for the classic, paternalistic approach to health care, in which patients are passive recipients of care delivered at a hospital or a physician's office during episodes of illness or injury.

Increasingly, people want to be treated as partners of their health care providers, with an active role in managing their wellness, both before they come into contact with a health care organization and in their return to health afterward. As part of this decisive shift in the classic health delivery paradigm, more and more people are actively seeking out other sources of health care information than traditional providers. Patients are now much more informed about treatment options than in the past and much more aggressive in pursuing them.

Technology has been a catalyst of both this craving for health care information and the ability to satisfy it. With mass market adoption of the Internet, the growing number of health- and wellness-related web sites gives people easy access to enormous quantities of health care information. They are, however, left with the task of sorting fact from fiction. Health care providers who wish to serve their communities thus have an additional obligation today of ensuring that the community as a whole, and not just their own patients, has access to timely, accurate, and relevant health care information.

This chapter describes the development of an integrated system for taking health information out into the community. By forming nontraditional partnerships and through the use of constantly evolving technologies, SHC is setting the stage for a new era in health care delivery.

Scottsdale as a Site for Health Care Innovation

SHC, a not-for-profit organization with a community-based board of directors, was created in 1962 to meet the health care needs of the Scottsdale, Arizona, region, a thriving community enjoying explosive growth. Scottsdale and the surrounding area's population of more than 500,000, spread across twenty-three zip codes, is projected to grow to more than 600,000 by 2001. There are high percentages of young families, empty nesters, Hispanics, and seniors. The median age of the population is thirty-eight years, and the average annual household income is $52,000, but there is also a significant number of underserved residents. Community health programming needs are different for each of the region's demographic groups, but on average Scottsdale is an informed and affluent community whose residents want to be partners with their health care providers.

At the core of SHC are two acute care hospitals with 510 medical-surgical beds, 16 rehabilitation beds, and 60 skilled nursing beds. Together, the two facilities offer a full range of services, including Level 1 trauma, obstetrics, general and specialized surgery, acute and long-term care, diagnostics, and rehabilitation. SHC also includes SHC FamilyCare, a network of primary care physicians located in neighborhoods throughout the greater Scottsdale area, and Scottsdale Health Care Home Health Services.

Partnering with the Community

To be successful in health care today, health care organizations must be perceived as caring about their customers. In part, this entails putting customer service first, above cutting costs and efficient resource management. For example, as an expression of its commitment to community health, all of the proceeds from SHC Foundation's major fundraising events since 1990 have gone to establishing formal community health education programs through the Community Health Education Department. Programs are aimed at improving longevity and the quality of life, focusing on individuals who are most at risk for lifestyle-related illness and injury. Wellness and prevention activities are key elements of these programs, which, following the life stage approach, begin in elementary school and extend to the senior years.

At the same time, accessibility to services is also a central feature of putting the customer first. As people become more familiar with information and communication technologies, they are increasingly frustrated by systems that do not use them to improve service. When a busy working mother needs advice on child development, she will remember both the health care provider who frustrates her by holding office hours only during the day and using an answering service during her lunch hour, and the health care provider who allows her access to information anytime she needs it. She will do business with the provider who makes access easy and provides the information she needs, when she needs it. The SHC competitive positioning strategy is thus to put the care of patients first, adapting its business organization and operations to their expectations and culture. In the process, SHC forges a relationship that earns customer loyalty.

Because it faces competition from a number of other large health care–oriented organizations in its region, partnerships have become an important element of SHC's competitive strategy. SHC approaches partnership with the community in three ways. First, it focuses on the needs of constituents. It works at creating the recognition in their minds that the SHC organization is so concerned about who they are, who their families are, and what their lifestyles are that there is no second thought on their part about who to call when they have a health question, concern, or problem. Becoming indispensable to its customers is the key to SHC's positioning strategy.

Second, SHC has established partnerships with schools, churches, service organizations, neighborhood developments, and other community groups to bring health and wellness education closer to home and work. It holds annual vision and hearing screenings in Scottsdale's schools, focus groups and an area-wide church survey to determine health concerns of city residents, risk appraisals, family safety programs, fitness programs, and free health education seminars and health screenings. In addition to improving the health of the community, these programs leave an impression that SHC is the community's resource for health and wellness.

Third, SHC has given customers access to alternative forms of health care information, such as a telephone-based information system, a technologically advanced health information center, and multimedia kiosks. By offering tailored educational programming and interactive health education through such avenues, customers have the opportunity to become active participants in their health. And with the widespread use of Internet and intranet technologies in the not-too-distant future, direct access to the health care organization will become even more the norm.

Building an Information Technology Foundation

Tying traditional and new forms of health care delivery together through technology that provides information throughout SHC is a key to successfully delivering customer-oriented health care. The integration of clinical and administrative data regarding the population whose health is being managed is central to changing the way health care is delivered. It is not enough just to gather segmented pieces of information on a patient during a single encounter with the managing organization. Discrete bits of information must be integrated into a lifetime health history of the customer, at all points of service across the enterprise. Documentation of all encounters a customer has with SHC—whether at the hospital, the physician's office, at home, over the Internet, or over the telephone—is paramount. Furthermore, by integrating its database of encounter information with other sources, such as employers or insurance companies, SHC can ensure that it has the most up-to-date demographic information on its customers.

SHC has partnered with Atlanta-based HBO & Company to provide health care software and networking systems that will build the foundation necessary to share information across the organization in support of redesigning SHC's health care services delivery system. Its access management strategy uses sophisticated technology to enable customers to access health services easily and cost-effectively. In addition, such a strategy provides the ability to know who SHC's customers are when they come into contact with any point of service in the organization.

For example, because Mr. Jones is a known customer to SHC, when his primary care physician refers him to the hospital to have tests run, he does not have to complete the usual paperwork on who he is and what his medical history is. That information is already in his electronic patient record. What this means for Mr. Jones is seamless access to care, resulting in positive perceptions of the health care organization, greater customer satisfaction and loyalty, and increased efficiency. Essentially, what Scottsdale did was to link all its customer interface activities through its internal information highway. The next step is to extend access management strategy to the community by providing tools directly to consumer households.

Then customers can participate actively in their care and partner with SHC in lifestyle management and wellness planning.

In 1997, SHC formed an alliance with the developers of DC Ranch, an 8,300–acre master planned community of forty-five hundred homes now under construction in the rugged peaks of the McDowell Mountains in north Scottsdale. SHC was selected as the preferred health care provider, based on its strong community reputation for quality service, its longevity in Scottsdale, commitment to technology, and long-standing community health education programming for the community, as well as its progress toward establishing an electronic link to the health enterprise.

The benefits to SHC in this partnership are twofold: using information technology to create routine interactive relationships with this young, growing community so that people there are more likely to turn to SHC when they need more intensive health care services, and the opportunity to create a showcase environment using technology to promote healthy lifestyles.

The developer of DC Ranch, Phoenix-based DMB and Associates, was founded in 1984 as a real estate development firm, and has grown to become a diversified investment company with interests in real estate, manufacturing, and business endeavors, although real estate remains the core of its focus. Its projects are of the highest quality, enhancing the surroundings and ensuring thoughtful, responsible development in the community. DMB is committed to an environment where people needing health care assistance will not have to get into a car but rather can communicate quickly with their care provider through the community intranet (RanchNet). To obtain preferred health care organization status at DC Ranch, SHC has committed to extending health care technology to the household. This will be accomplished by deploying HealthDesk Corporation's HealthDesk Online personal health and care management software on the health care consumer's home computer.

US West, the DC Ranch technology partner, will establish "fiber to the curb" at each of the home sites in DC Ranch, with the equivalent of greater than Integrated Services Digital Network (ISDN) connection capability, giving SHC the intranet infrastructure needed to provide the high-tech alternatives to health care discussed here: virtual kiosks, consumer-based health management software, and direct on-line links from the household to the provider.

DC Ranch, which has become Scottsdale's model for extending health care technology to the consumer household, was developed on the three principles of education, wellness, and technology. The goal is to make it easy for health care consumers to obtain information over an intranet and other centrally located sources like the Health Resource Center, so they have an opportunity to live healthier lifestyles and make more informed choices about how to use health care services most effectively. SHC programs embrace advanced technology as well as education with all aspects of the community, including the planned school system, K–12, and the adult education provided by the local university on site. In addition to easy access to health care, the approximately fifteen thousand residents of DC Ranch will be able to walk to the grocery store on neighborhood trails, enjoy the desert evening chatting with neighbors on the front porch, or step out their back door to take a hike through the preserved desert terrain.

DC Ranch will offer acres of open space and breathtaking views wherever the resident is: whether in a residential neighborhood, at one of the many parks and golf courses, or at one of the schools, churches, medical facilities, or retail stores. The premise is to mix the most advanced technology with old-fashioned values to increase the quality of life. It has been called a "back to the future" style community. It draws a comparison between DC Ranch and the movie that shows life in a 1950s small town where teenagers ride home from school on skateboards that hover a few inches off the ground, then sit down with their families for a well-balanced dinner. Instead of hovercrafts, the technologies of choice at DC Ranch will be the Internet and virtual reality, and the well-balanced meals may be prepared by chefs at the Health Resource Center for today's families on the go.

When development of the Health Resource Center is completed in October 1999, it will combine a number of health and wellness components. DC Ranch residents will be able to conduct a video teleconference with a nutritionist or other clinicians, schedule an appointment with their primary care physician through the health care concierge (the health care professional staffing the center), attend educational or fitness classes, or get health information from a touch-screen kiosk.

The Health Resource Center is about lifestyle. It is designed to be an overall community gathering place where DC Ranch residents can come to relax, eat a healthy meal, and get the latest health information. If Mr. Jones, for example, were a resident of DC Ranch, there are a number of opportunities he would have to live a healthier lifestyle. He might start his day with a brisk walk at 6 A.M. with his walking club, then end up at the Health Resource Center for a healthy breakfast of decaffeinated coffee and a bran muffin. Midmorning, he might attend a yoga class, followed by a low-fat sub for lunch. And in the afternoon, Mr. Jones could attend a cooking demonstration where he would learn how to prepare "Heart Saviour" recipes that have been developed using good nutrition, with less fat, salt, and cholesterol. These are just examples of the number of things that will be going on in the Health Resource Center in addition to walk-in information and the health care concierge, designed to be the community's resource for health-related questions, issues, and needs. This position, modeled after the typical hotel concierge, is a community asset, there to provide needed information and service related to healthy lifestyles, as well as disease management information.

The Health Resource Center offers a broader range of services, but residents do not have to go there for their health lifestyle information and interaction. HealthDesk is another big piece of community health access at DC Ranch. The HealthDesk OnLine private web site offers a ten-million-page virtual library of health education resources, health-related articles from publications ranging from the

New York Times to the *Journal of the American Medical Association* (*JAMA*), and reference materials. An expansion of the symptom triage handbook, the HEALTHWISE Knowledgebase, also is available on-line to provide subscribers and their families with a powerful decision support tool.

By giving DC Ranch residents access to the many features of HealthDesk OnLine—a virtual health care library, interactive self-assessment tools, on-line bulletin boards, and sponsored forums—SHC is in effect giving DC Ranch residents an alternative to the Health Resource Center. In addition, DC Ranch provides the infrastructure for a direct connection through the intranet to the health care concierge at the Health Resource Center as well as to SHC's staff primary care physicians.

Justifying Community Access

SHC has chosen to be involved in community access programs like DC Ranch that do not generate direct revenue because it brands SHC health services offerings and its commitment to a large group of potential customers whose loyalty will be won based on access to information and the health care services SHC is perceived to be able to provide. Building a new customer base is difficult because in today's consumer-driven marketplace, health care providers have to prove themselves constantly. The cost of deploying health care technology in a start-up community like DC Ranch is accepted by SHC as a necessary expenditure in pursuit of twenty thousand new, and potentially very loyal, customers, critical if SHC is to beat its competition.

Further, loyal customers are far more supportive when they see their health care provider as their partner. If SHC makes enough good impressions in the minds of its customers, it will create a trusting relationship with them. With DC Ranch, SHC hopes to provide so many positive health care encounters through a number of different media that a customer will have no second thoughts about seeking health care services from it and will not go looking elsewhere. SHC aims to make itself indispensable.

Finally, customer loyalty is dependent on the age-old concept too long ignored by health care providers: know your customers and make their culture your culture. For too many years, health care organizations have expected customers to adapt to their systems. Now, health care organizations are beginning to realize that to stay in the game, they must adapt their systems to customer demands. To compete, they must provide health care that caters to a number of demographic groups, from generation Xers to the baby boomers to the Medicare population. Health care organizations must be agile in their approach to health care service delivery in order to be able to deliver services in forms that each of these populations will accept. No longer can we follow the adage, "Build it and they will come."

Evolving Role of the Health Care Provider

Understanding why SHC has evolved from a traditional provider of acute health care services to a provider of customer-focused health where healthy lifestyles are the norm provides a rationale for its involvement with DC Ranch and support for HealthDesk. It also illuminates some of the limitations of traditional health care and how new technologies can help overcome them.

Critical Paths

Like any other major health care organization, SHC was in the business of providing care primarily for patients with acute health problems. Also like other health care organizations, this care extended across a continuum of services—skilled nursing, testing, home care—that were delivered in a segmented rather than an integrated manner, over critical paths that managed the acute needs of a patient on a day-to-day basis. There was no way to manage an episode of care across multiple settings, much less across the lifetime of a health care customer. Over time, case management programs were put in place to manage the patient better throughout his or her episode, but the bottom line was the same: no coordination across the lifetime of the patient or beyond the patient's release from the hospital, home health service, or long-term care facility.

Community Health Education

In an effort to look beyond the four walls of the hospital, SHC initiated the "Take Good Care of Yourself" community health education series in 1989. The programs center on structured classes, seminars, and information centers where people are offered disease-specific health prevention information, as well as wellness screenings. SHC also offered a variety of information services through its teleservices organization, which provides physician referrals, registration for education offerings, and information on general health topics and specific disease states. The program is designed to encourage callers to obtain important information regarding any health topic in which they may be interested.

In addition to teleservices, SHC manages chronic disease processes through a telemanagement center, coordinated through SHC Home Health Services. Upon referral to the program by their physician, patients with diabetes, congestive heart failure, and chronic obstructive pulmonary disease are managed by a registered nurse over the telephone, who initiates and monitors treatment plans using preapproved guidelines and care criteria. (Other diseases will be added as needed.) As problems arise, patients are directed to an appropriate level of care: a home health nurse, a visit to the physician's office or emergency room, or, in the worst case, calling 911. This has been a successful program both financially and from the perspective of patient and physician satisfaction. HealthTouch gives community members open access to an automated system that provides information on more than one thousand common health topics. For example, callers can find information on high blood cholesterol, cancer signs, and how to quit smoking. The automated system, which can be accessed twenty-four hours a day and has bilingual capabilities, includes recordings on women's concerns, including breast self-examination, breast cancer, contraception methods, estrogen replacement therapy, hysterectomy, mammography, and menopause. The information can be customized for a variety of uses, such as providing information on SHC's health education programs or local health topics. At any time during business hours, the caller can exit the program and reach a teleservices operator; off-hours are handled by an automated call distribution system. The information received can be printed and sent to the callers.

Neighborhood Initiatives

SHC also brings health care to the community through thirteen FamilyCare sites, which offer primary, pediatric, and obstetric care to its service area. The evolution of the sites began in the summer of 1995, and planned-for expansion will take place as needs are identified. SHC partners with six master plan communities in its service area—DC Ranch being the most technologically advanced of the six—to provide health care and lifestyle education to residents. Services offered include on-site education, seminars and screenings in community centers, community CPR classes, health risk appraisals, walking clubs, and health membership programs.

Community Collaborative

SHC is a member of a community collaborative called LINKS. This is strictly a volunteer organization and receives its funding from its participants, which include the City of Scottsdale, the Scottsdale Chamber of Commerce, the Scottsdale Unified School District, Scottsdale Community College, SHC, the YMCA, the Boys and Girls Clubs, and the Scottsdale Prevention Institute.

LINKS is a growing network of individuals and organizations committed to sharing responsibilities and resources to create a community that is safe, healthy, and productive for children, adults, and families. It is not another program or agency; rather, it provides a framework for sharing and coordinating goals, strategies, responsibilities, and accountability among existing programs and agencies.

LINKS grew out of a growing realization that Scottsdale is not immune to the many ills that make the lives of families, youths, and adults challenging, difficult, and sometimes desperate. The pattern of discrete, fragmented social, economic, and health care services that prevails nationwide also has roots in Scottsdale. The needs, however, cross over the boundaries of the organizations charged with providing them, and go beyond the resources of any single organization. The vision of LINKS is to reverse this fragmentation by working together as a total community.

New Approaches

SHC's FamilyCare facilities, community health education, health call center system, and telemanagement program are all traditional community outreach programs that bring health and wellness information to its customers. Although these are useful sources of general health information, today's consumers want quick, convenient access to accurate information from a respected community health care provider to help them make health lifestyle choices for themselves and their families. Through community focus groups and a community survey conducted for it by a well-known national survey and polling firm, SHC learned that health care consumers want a "one-stop-shop" approach to health care and health information—and they want that stop to be within a five- to nine-mile radius of their home.

Putting Technology to Work

These findings have been a driving force in meeting the demands of increasingly sophisticated consumers. SHC's newest approaches to health and wellness programs are designed with these consumers in mind. For example, SHC put in one of its hospitals a health information center that includes a multitude of resources on disease entities, wellness, and prevention that go beyond traditional periodicals and books to include CD-ROMs, software packages, and connections to Internet sites.

SHC is exploring ways to deliver such technology to its community through touch-screen kiosks. In doing so, it is working with a state-of-the-art kiosk developer, First Wave Software Innovation, in breaking information boundaries. By providing economical, reliable, and self-updating touch-screen technology, SHC is looking for a fast, easy-to-use, multifeatured offering that provides a positive return on investment. SHC is also evaluating how to take this type of service into other community sites, including shopping malls and mobile vans. As with its teleservices, SHC believes that the kiosk technology will give health care consumers information to make better-informed choices regarding health care. As an alternative to the telephone as the technological means of communication between the consumer and SHC, the kiosks employ interactive multimedia, such as video and virtual reality, to provide information.

Consumers can walk up to the touch-screen kiosks and have online access to current disease-specific information, read biographical data on physicians, "walk" through an examination room, and view video clips on health topics that give them answers to virtually all their health care questions. Kiosk technology has already merged with telephones, enabling users to link directly with the Teleservices Department for further information. The natural next progression for kiosk technology surely is convergence with the Internet.

Managing the Health of a Population

With a number of traditional and nontraditional community access programs that give the people of greater Scottsdale easier and more cost-efficient access to health care and health information, the next step is to begin managing the health of the population. One way to do this is to have customers complete a self-assessment of their health on a yearly or semiyearly basis using nationally recognized health assessment tools. SHC can use such customer-authored data to monitor health status and send periodic health-related information or appointment reminders. For example, if Mrs. Jones is fifty years old and her self-assessment says it has been two years since her last mammogram, SHC can send her a reminder notice and encourage her to schedule an appointment for service. Taking that one step further, if SHC can manage the health statistics of its customer population over time, it can design programs and services to meet their evolving needs better.

To deliver population management most effectively, information technology must be used to automate processes so that when a customer provides information—whether through a self-assessment, through an encounter with the teleservices information center, or via e-mail—the organization can respond in a timely manner. The ultimate goal at DC Ranch, as well as with other community-focused initiatives, is to integrate appropriate customer-authored data into SHC's data repository so that information becomes part of the customer's lifetime health record. This will give SHC health care professionals a powerful, interactive management tool that will enable them to pinpoint specific problems and focus interventions on patients who are experiencing problems or need specific support. Ultimately, SHC believes, customers will complete routine assessments such as pre-op histories on-line at home and then submit them electronically to be reviewed and validated, after which they will be stored as part of their medical records.

Emerging Technologies in Health Care

The future of automated health care delivery lies in the Internet and intranet technologies. A growing body of focused study and survey data suggests that a large number of consumers are interested in and willing to accept delivery of health care via on-line services. Moreover, the potential of health care delivery using the Internet is a reality, and it will grow as the number of households with computers and Internet access grows over the next decade. With the evolution of new technologies like network computers and Web TV, the cost to the average household continues to become more attractive.

Approximately 40 percent of households (nearly 40 million) in the United States have computers, with penetration projected to increase to 50 percent of all homes by the year 2000. In addition, 70 percent of these households report owning a modem. Of modem owners, 46 percent subscribe to an on-line service, and an additional 26 percent use the Internet through another type of gateway, such as an office, educational institution, or gateway provider (American Management Association and Tierney & Partners, 1997).

Personal use of the Internet is rising rapidly. Activity at the numerous health, medical, and wellness sites on the Internet today indicates a thirst for health information by on-line consumers. A recent study of Internet users found that more than 80 percent of current users were interested in tapping into health-related information ("Experts Explore . . . ," 1996). However, many consumers are confused by the sheer quantity of health information on the Internet, and most are concerned about the quality of what is available.

Over the next decade, the Internet will play a pivotal role as networked consumer health information systems change health care just as profoundly as the economic engines and incentives of managed care did. One job of SHC as an agile health care provider is to help consumers sift through the myriad health information sites on the Internet, so that they get reliable information. SHC plans to do this through HealthDesk Online. This software product will enable SHC to unleash knowledge, form health-related communities, and create customer loyalty.

SHC will leverage HealthDesk OnLine to harness the power of the Internet and provide a confidential information and resource link between consumers and the SHC system. HealthDesk, designed for use in general populations to offer more efficient forms of demand management and customer service, provides a combination of security, consumer control, confidentiality, and access to reliable Internet information resources. In addition to providing customers with general health and wellness information and tracking, HealthDesk Online will give them connectivity to physicians employed by SHC, as well as HealthDesk's private web site. Encrypted information is transmitted over any Internet service provider the consumer may have.

By providing HealthDesk to its customers (the software resides on the subscriber's desktop computer), SHC empowers them to play an active, and interactive, role in their health care. At the same time, it creates an opportunity for customers to partner with SHC in cost and utilization management. Customers will be able to track personal and family history and health-related activities. They also will be able to obtain reliable information on exercise, nutrition, vital statistics, medications, personal expenditures, and physician visits.

In addition to health care information, HealthDesk Online provides secure two-way message exchange between SHC customers and SHC physicians, health plans, and employers. This provides them with a high-tech way to ask questions and potentially receive answers at any time. It gives SHC the opportunity to supplement or supplant existing paper- and telephone-based communications, resulting in administrative savings and increased customer satisfaction. SHC case managers also can use the messaging function in managing their high-risk clients.

Conclusion

In today's health care market, the only way for providers to stay alive and to be competitive is to be innovative. To be innovative requires that an organization be flexible, have an ability to adjust to change, and routinely incorporate breakthrough thinking. Agility provides a comprehensive context for developing innovative health care initiatives. For this reason, SHC has sought partners on the cutting edge of technology. In concert with its partners, it acquires the tools to keep SHC the leader in its market. With the shrinking reimbursement being experienced in heavily managed care markets, health systems have had to devote far more resources to enlarging their share of the market. For that reason, SHC adopted a community access focus using creative techniques and relying on flexibility of design. SHC is keeping pace with marketplace change through its leadership in designing programs for its community's varied neighborhoods, in the process making SHC indispensable to its customers.

7

Information as a Competitive Health Care Resource

Leanne Kaiser Carlson, Scott Hendrickson

We live in the midst of an information technology explosion that is altering every aspect of health care delivery. The combination of steeply declining costs and increasing power has made computing ubiquitous, and this has made possible a spectacular array of new medical applications. Implantable microdevices, on-line global knowledge bases, artificial intelligence software, and an expanding array of increasingly sophisticated visualization technologies are reshaping health care. Information technologies enable more effective resource allocations, optimize clinical practice patterns, and make possible learning on demand in the context of real-time clinical practice.

Intelligent devices monitor patient conditions and alert physicians when parameters exceed threshold values. Some suggest treatment modifications for physician approval or modification, after which they communicate the new instructions to the patient unit for action. Clinicians test diagnostic assumptions and planned courses of therapeutic action in simulated environments prior to treating actual patients. Providers and patients interact through video links that allow surgical, as well as diagnostic, procedures to be performed remotely.

Computerization has already influenced nearly every aspect of life for the average American, from shopping and banking to workplace automation and security systems. Time spent on computerized games and Internet access is significantly displacing leisure time that used to be devoted to television viewing. Today, the average new car contains more computing power than was on board the *Apollo* spacecraft that carried astronauts to and from the moon (Olson, 1996). Microprocessors control the engine, transmission, brakes, suspension, lights, heating/cooling, audio system, dashboard displays, and communication. Yet for most people, this wonder of information automation—in which the value of the electronics exceeds the value of the steel—is still just a car. So it will be in health care, as myriad new information technologies work transparently behind the scenes to support new ways of performing business and clinical functions smarter, faster, cheaper, and therefore better.

Such embedded information technology dramatically enhances agility as people and organizations learn in new ways, perform work through virtual teams and real-time interactive collaborations, deliver care over geographic and other boundaries, benefit from time and financial efficiencies, and harness technology to increase effective intelligence and capability. This chapter explores each of these dynamics of agility, their current application in health care, and some examples of the information infrastructure that need to be put in place to realize the benefits they promise. The software technologies and techniques described allow readers to visualize a pathway from the all-too-easy accumulation of massive quantities of data, to the more difficult integration and transformation of data into information, to the very challenging conversion of information into knowledge through analysis, including emerging capabilities for automated information analysis.

Accelerating Learning

Health care organizations increasingly compete with each other on marginal differences in cost. As managed care pressures drive discounting and force changes in resource allocation, competitors must match these discounts or differentiate themselves through superior outcomes. Excellence in knowledge capture and information management is the key to a differentiation strategy based on cost-effective outcomes improvement.

Health care is among the most information-intensive industries. The total amount of information in the field of medicine now doubles every eighteen months. By contrast, it took fifteen hundred years for the West to double the amount of information it had inherited from classical Greek and Roman medical practitioners. Information technologies, from Gutenberg's printing press and the first academic journals to word processors and the Internet, drive the rate of information growth. This, in turn, drives the rate of social change, placing constantly increasing demands on individuals and institutions who must deal with this information.

Nurses, for example, spend approximately 50 percent of their time recording data in the patient chart. Researchers create new drugs, new therapies, and new practice management techniques and accumulate a flood tide of data for physicians and administrators. Yet as Ozbolt suggests (1997), for all the charting, the research, the clinical studies, and the data collection, there is little ability to answer such obviously valuable questions as these:

- Which care practices are associated with the best balance of length of stay, cost of care, and patient outcomes?
- Under different configurations of resource allocation, what happens to problems identified, actions taken, and outcomes achieved?
- Which care practices are ineffective or even harmful and therefore should be discontinued or changed?
- Which care practices are associated with such substantially better patient outcomes that they merit the greater resources they require?

Studies such as *The Dartmouth Atlas of Health Care* (Wennberg and Cooper, 1998) demonstrate that practice patterns vary substantially. In the most recent *Atlas*, carotid endarterectomy shows a sevenfold variation, with a high of 7.1 per 1,000 Medicare enrollees in Houma, Louisiana, to lows of 0.98 per 1,000 in Honolulu and 1.04 per 1,000 in Idaho Falls. Similarly, back surgery varies from 1.3 to 7.6 per 1,000 Medicare enrollees; and the rate of radical prostatectomy varies ninefold, from 0.05 to 4.9 per 1,000. In some years, mastectomy versus lumpectomy has varied thirty-three–fold, even though women survive equally long with lumpectomy as with mastectomy. Even the chance of dying in a hospital varies radically, from 20 percent of all Medicare deaths in some regions of the country to more than 50 percent in other regions after adjusting for age, sex, and racial differences.

To identify best practice patterns and answer effectiveness and efficiency questions, data must be defined, collected, stored, accessed, and used differently than they are now. Additionally, new data elements that go beyond the Uniform Hospital Discharge Data Set must be included. Best practices can then be benchmarked both within and among organizations.

Data Warehousing

The data warehouse is a powerful new software tool that is evolving rapidly, driven by the need to integrate vast quantities of data into operational-level decision processes.

One of the foundations of personal human intelligence is our ability to recall facts, events, and concepts and structure them in the context of current situations to identify similarities, patterns, and potential consequences. Analogously, a key to organizational intelligence is the ability to access and structure an organization's memory. The data warehouse, which performs these functions, is an important technology for an organization wishing to develop more sophisticated and effective decision and process structures.

Many organizations rely on the personal memory of a few key individuals in the organization—or worse, chance and ad hoc methods—for maintaining organizational intelligence. However, with the emerging technologies in information organization and storage and the growing availability of mature on-line analytical processing (OLAP) tools, an organization can make a great deal of its collective memory available to nontechnical users. We will explain briefly the components of the data warehouse and its use and give some examples of how health care organizations are using their data warehouses.

The "products" of the data warehouse are answers to three questions: What happened? Why did it happen? and What will happen in the future? To answer these questions in ways that increase efficiency, a data warehousing project must effectively implement three data warehouse components: a structure and standard form for abstracting and organizing data, physical infrastructure including hardware and software to facilitate storage and access to the data, and tools that will allow nontechnical users to query and analyze the data.

To support these tools, the data abstracting structures must be chosen to facilitate decisions and learning around the core objectives specific to the business of the organization. Employees will need to have access to the right information at the time when, and from the place where, learning and decision making occur. Access must be available across geographical boundaries and computing platforms.

The challenge of connectivity across geography, computational platforms, and organizations is being met with the increasing maturity of the Internet; the prevalence, low cost, and increasing capability of thin clients such as Java-enabled web browsers; and the security and versatility of three-tiered client-server architectures based on CORBA (common object request broker architecture) and other open standards. As these tools mature, they bring higher capabilities, integration, and connectivity at costs increasingly justifiable by large returns on investment. Furthermore, the complications of connectivity and security can be hidden from users, allowing them to focus on getting answers to their questions.

An organization's hardware and software infrastructure must match the scale of the organization's memory requirements and accessibility needs. Finally, the data analysis tools must provide a comprehensive set of standard reports and the capability for non-technical users to build complex queries and generate custom reports. Emerging technologies that facilitate this process include sophisticated custom query and analysis tools and learning systems that make use of genetic algorithms and artificial neural networks.

Data abstraction and encoding or the data warehouse scheme must be chosen to support an organization's key business processes and facilitate strategic decisions. This requires information technology staff to have a deep understanding of the business objectives of the organization and how each business process supports these objectives.

When mature and effective processes are supported by appropriate data abstraction and encoding, a high level of data integration combined with powerful reporting tools enables sophisticated organizational intelligence. This ability to analyze and create a complete picture of costs, resources, and the interactions of processes across the entire organization results in the strength and flexibility necessary for a competitive position in the marketplace and the self-understanding required to create an agile strategy for the future.

Organizations are choosing to integrate a broadening array of data in their data warehouses. For example, Omni Health Care, a health management organization (HMO) in northern California serving 130,000 members, aggregates data from, and provides access to these data to, five groups of users:

- Actuary staff can review companywide costs for medical supplies, services, and pharmaceuticals. This allows competitive decision making and contracting.
- Marketing personnel can evaluate the demographics of Omni's membership and measure the success of marketing efforts.

- Membership accounting staff can track payments and produce reports.
- Provider group staff can better match member demand to providers' capabilities and analyze provider expenses for competitive contract negotiation.
- Medical management staff can compare internal practices with the industry's best practices. This improves strategic decision making and provides a competitive advantage.

Omni has integrated this information under one OLAP tool that allows users to create custom queries and reports that can show correlations across business groups. This high level of integration allows a new kind of agile intelligence.

Learning in an Agile Organization

Agile organizations both learn effectively from their own information and can tap into an extended universe of knowledge bases, people, and educational materials and learn on demand, as needed in the context of clinical practice. Such learning supports agility by improving both efficiency and effectiveness. It delivers information conveniently and in the appropriate amount, and does so in real time, when the relevance and potential for retention are highest.

One health care organization at the forefront of such agile learning is the University of Iowa, home of the "Virtual Hospital." Here, the goal is to create a web-based system that integrates continuing education directly into the provider's work flow. Key terms in the computerized patient record (CPR) link to relevant multimedia educational resources. Physicians access information directly through the CPR and receive fractional continuing medical education (CME) credit (D'Alessandro and others, 1996). The concept of a fractional or granular CME issued in this way is new and must be approved by medical schools, as well as accepted by state medical licensing agencies. But in industry generally, such approval is consistent with current trends in continuing education, reflecting the need for agility in all organizations.

Simulation adds another dimension to agility by enabling learning to occur outside the constraints and consequences of physical reality. Although simulations of increasing complexity have become routine in other fields, such as engineering, finance, and physics, simulation is just now beginning to be used in health care.

CAE Electronics, whose core competency is flight training simulators, recently developed a patient simulator for anesthesia training. This includes a mannequin that breathes through servo-controlled lungs, exhibits palpable pulses at the carotid and radial arteries, and even has a simulated twitch for the assessment of neuromuscular blockade. The mannequin responds to seventy-five different drugs, interfaces with anesthesia machines and other monitoring equipment, and models twenty-eight critical events, such as anaphylaxis, aspiration, hemorrhage, and coronary constriction.

Dozens of other simulations model the behavior of organs, the efficacy of drug and other therapies, disease processes, the results of surgical and other procedures, as well as a variety of business and administrative concerns. These simulations, and others like them, are currently used for training and surely will be used for credentialing purposes in the near future, but inevitably such tools will soon be used in actual practice as well. For example, a computer simulation is being used by United Network for Organ Sharing to allocate organs for transplants nationwide.

Virtual Teams and Collaborative Work

The agile health care organization reinvents work processes, communication, and roles. People move seamlessly through organizational and geographic boundaries and work in an environment of cross-functional teams, opportunistic outsourcing, mobility, decentralized decision making, and virtual arrangements. Technology enables this agility by facilitating instantaneous access to information from any location. Medical records, diagnostic images, lab results, verbal and written communications, ancillary service requests, claims submissions, and other data may be exchanged to coordinate care across the health care continuum.

Internet technologies are perhaps the single greatest advance in this area, enabling communication across platforms and standardizing protocols for information display and access. Industry experts estimate that within five years, more than half of the medical records in the United States and Europe will be browser based (Gage, 1996).

At the same time, the sheer volume of data being collected enables sophisticated prediction and modeling of alternative therapies and outcomes. Such is the case at the Duke Clinical Research Institute, where a multivariate database contains thirty years of detailed clinical heart attack data, painstakingly registered by doctors, nurses, and researchers. Every spasm, every chemical released into the bloodstream, every treatment, and every outcome is etched in silicon. Physicians across the world dial into this system, enter clinical and other relevant information about their particular patient's case, and receive recommendations for treatment based on tens of thousands of similar patients and their responses in the past (Ramo, 1996).

Physicians, staff, managers, strategic partners, and clients are increasingly demanding faster, more up-to-date, and more comprehensive access to information. Therefore, a comprehensive on-line strategy must include plans for managing technology and content intended for three audiences: employees and staff, strategic business partners, and clients. Each group has its own set of expectations from content and technology and its own set of security requirements.

The first group, employees and staff, are those targeted by the traditional intranet, comprising the on-line tools and information accessed through web technologies (web or intranet servers and thin clients, such as browsers communicating through a local area or wide area network), but available only to an internal audience. Usually intranets are protected from public access by being physically disconnected from the Internet or by software called a firewall that filters network traffic.

Intranet users expect up-to-date information to be available day after day. They depend on this information to make decisions, effectively provide and support products and services, and make them aware of changes in the organization. Security should be robust but transparent to intranet users.

Currently organizations use intranets to accomplish these purposes:

- Broadcast and publish internally
- Share corporate knowledge and support
- Search for data and information
- Support group calendaring (after the fact) and scheduling (before the fact)
- Access information from a known source
- Edit and manage documents in a group
- Manage projects in a distributed work group
- Access remote or distributed applications
- Support mobile workers

The second group, strategic business partners, are those targeted by the extranet. These are the business partners with whom an organization must communicate securely and do business with regularly—for example: an insurer that provides on-line claims submission, or a medical equipment supplier authorized to fill a standing order automatically when supplies fall below a predefined level. As with the intranet, communications are accomplished through web technologies. In addition, strategic partners are often linked to an organization through secure connections, either privately leased or, increasingly, through encryption and authentication using a virtual private network (VPN) over the public Internet lines. Typically strategic partners need regular and secure access to very specific just-in-time information.

Currently organizations use extranets to do the following:

- Process orders with just-in-time suppliers to reduce inventory costs and shorten lead times
- Share product and service information and support
- Transmit and process forms for claims, orders, and so forth
- Provide point-of-service data entry capabilities
- Communicate across geographical boundaries
- Rapidly process business transactions

The third group targeted by a comprehensive on-line strategy is current and prospective clients. Clients access information and tools over the Internet using a web browser. A typical Internet site contains information on services and facilities intended for the public, as in a traditional print brochure, on-line services such as the physician referral applications, or health information databases found on many hospital web sites, and may also offer information and services that a client can purchase on-line. Examples include consulting services such as those available from the Ernst & Young web site (http://ernie.ey.com) or products such as books from Amazon.com (http://www.amazon.com).

Risks and Challenges

Along with the many benefits of on-line communications comes a new set of risks and challenges, which must be met with a new way of thinking about information, information access, security, and technology. Traditionally, a health care organization's information services (IS) or marketing department is responsible for on-line content and technologies. Often a web presence is a grass-roots effort and not driven by a comprehensive on-line strategy consistent with the core business objectives of an organization. Without integration into the overall business strategy and clear business objectives, an intranet, extranet, or Internet presence will fail to support business processes and provide no competitive advantage.

In order to meet the challenges of implementing a comprehensive on-line strategy, an organization must invest in the process and personnel to support three necessary functions (DePalma and others, 1996):

- *On-line strategy team*. This team has the responsibly for articulating, disseminating, and maintaining an ongoing on-line strategy consistent with the business objectives of the organization. It is important that the strategy group include members of the content and technology teams so that these teams have a deep understanding of business objectives and complete buy-in to the on-line strategy. It is important that this organization not be driven primarily by technology.
- *Content creation and maintenance team*. This team has the responsibility of planning for and driving the creation and maintenance of content targeted toward intranet, Internet, and extranet users. The actual creation of content is likely to happen at many levels and across the entire organization. It is this team's responsibility to coordinate and integrate content creation. Key members of this group must work closely with the strategy group.
- *Technology support team*. This is the domain of traditional IS. It is important for the technology support

team to include members of both the content and strategy teams so that these teams know what is technologically possible and the cost and time for new technology creation.

Content Strategy: Reshaping the Nature of Content

As information becomes more readily available, expectations of the type and comprehensiveness of information available and the speed with which it can be accessed are growing. Increasingly, customers expect to find product and service support—information they formerly got by talking on the telephone to a representative—on-line. Patients increasingly expect to find service, facility, and physician information through the web.

One reason for the rising expectations is that the volume of information can be many times larger than before, yet access can be simpler and faster than traditional means. For example, on-line a user can search a telephone book of the entire United States from a simple search screen. And unlike a traditional telephone book, the on-line system can be searched by state, partial names, and a host of other criteria. As storage capacity and analysis tools expand and mature, comprehensive, easily accessed content will be demanded by patients, employees, and partners.

With rising expectations comes a proliferation of information. One result is that information becomes less an asset to an organization than the knowledge and understanding of what to do with it. Information monopolies become less common while organizations succeed on knowing what to do with the information. Agile organizations will leverage their ability to use information to operate more efficiently and effectively and retain a competitive edge.

Technology Strategy

IS professionals regularly face the competing challenges to provide stable, continuous service and adapt to the rising demands and expectations of users by implementing new technologies. Many organizations face long and expensive technology upgrade projects because older systems either are incompatible with newer systems or cannot scale to meet increasing demand.

One strategy for dealing with these challenges is to minimize the number of proprietary components used in building information technology solutions. Components become "standard" through industry consensus, typically through a competitive, maturating process. Database engines implementing the current SQL (structured query language) standard, three-tier client-server system based on the CORBA standard, Java-based distributed applications, and a host of other open standards–based tools and components promise extendability and interoperability well beyond the capabilities of proprietary solutions.

Choosing technologies based on open standards increases the strength and flexibility of information technology solutions in these ways:

- Decreases an organization's dependence on key vendors
- Allows rapid adaptation to changing requirements as vendors offer mature tools and components
- Bases critical applications on proven technologies with broad capabilities
- Creates opportunities for systems that were originally constructed separately to become interoperable
- Provides opportunities to use cost-effective, commercially available solutions to integrate and update legacy systems

The level of connectivity and integration provided by on-line technologies is unprecedented. An organization willing to invest in content and personnel to provide system and data integration can achieve greater organizational intelligence than previously possible.

This will provide the agility necessary to remain competitive for years to come.

Extended Care Delivery

Information technology eliminates or reduces many barriers that have impeded agility in the past. Time barriers become less critical as communication occurs asynchronously, language barriers are countered with automatic translation applications, and geographic boundaries give way to high levels of interconnectivity that extend even into the home. As barriers such as time, language, and geography diminish, health care becomes a global business and the home once again becomes a primary health care delivery site.

Experiments with tele-home health are under way today. Kaiser Permanente, for example, uses tele-home health units with two-way videoconferencing, telephonic stethoscopes, and blood pressure cuffs for patients with chronic illnesses. Patients may access nurses using these units at any time of the day or night. Traditional home health visits complement these tele-home health consultations as appropriate. A study of this approach, scheduled to be formally released in 1998, suggests that such units are cost-effective and lead to improved patient outcomes and higher patient satisfaction.

HealthPartners in Minneapolis, Minnesota, uses similar technology for patients meeting specific criteria (see Exhibit 7.1). Early results show cost savings of 30 percent, half of which results from less need for inpatient hospitalization. With these and other applications in mind, it is no surprise that chief information officers, vice presidents of information systems, management information systems managers, and consultants identify access to on-line health information and services from the home as the most significant health care–related computer development affecting the average person in the next three years (Elliot, 1996).

Hundreds of thousands of patients and enrollees now depend on nurse advice lines with simple voice communication. Soon communication to physicians and other providers will be improved with

Exhibit 7.1. Criteria for Tele-Home Care Used by HealthPartners

Clinical Indications

Chronic disease in a state of decline:

- Congestive heart failure
- Chronic lung disease
- Diabetes
- Dementia
- Cancer

Operational Indications

Patients requiring two or more home care nursing visits per week

Patients who do not require "hands-on" care with each visit

Patients with an unreliable caregiver situation

Patients with poor compliance to instructions or medication use

Utilization Indications

Patients requiring frequent clinic visits (they are usually anxious)

Patients seen in the emergency room within the past two months

Patients hospitalized within the past six months

Source: Barry K. Baines, HealthPartners, Minneapolis, Minnesota.

two-way video directly into the home. Ultimately the capacity of such systems will be extended through remote instrumentation, diagnostics, and intelligence built directly into the patient units.

Massachusetts Institute of Technology (MIT), as well as the military, has demonstrated that it is possible to transmit to remote sites very fine physical movements, such as those required in surgery, using visual and manual technological "slaves." In the MIT case, visual, auditory, and mechanical information is relayed in two directions. A helmet worn by the surgeon (the visual master) controls a stereo camera system (the visual slave) at the surgical site. Images are then relayed back to the surgeon, who sees them either via the helmet or an adjacent screen. Similarly, as the surgeon manipulates pseudotools, this results in motion via a micromotion robot (the mechanical slave) that performs the actual surgery. A computer filters hand tremor and performs safety checks. For example, it would detect and impede rapid movement toward a delicate structure. Scaling of movement is also possible, enabling the surgeon to feel very fine forces that would normally be imperceptible and perform with precision as movements are scaled down by one to one hundred times.

Creating Efficiencies

The automation of and seamless access to information enables efficiencies of time and money, accomplished primarily through improved productivity, error reduction, lowered liability, and better communication.

Productivity improves through the automation of routine functions, leading to higher compliance, greater consistency, legibility, accuracy and timeliness of documentation, and decreased time spent obtaining, charting, and communicating redundant information. Researchers at Duke Family Medicine Center, for example, report savings of seven dollars per patient after the computerization of medical records in a large family practice setting (Wager, Ornstein, and Jenkins, 1997). Hospitals also are quantifying efficiencies. Pitt County Memorial Hospital in Greensboro, North Carolina, found that data management requires twenty-nine minutes less per nurse in a twelve-hour shift with the computerized system. At the same time, charting quality (as measured by eight indicators) improved from 62 percent to 95 percent, unplanned overtime decreased, unsupported reimbursement charges decreased, and the time required to do chart reviews for maintenance and nursing process audits decreased 50 percent (White and Hemby, 1997).

Error reduction contributes substantially to the financial and quality impact of information technology. The prevention of adverse drug events is one of the early and most dramatic areas for error reduction. Every year in the United States, approximately 200,000 people die because of adverse drug events, and the cost of these events to the health care system exceeds $76 billion annually

(Schneider, 1996a, p. 37). It is estimated that as much as 80 percent of these drug events can be prevented by alerting providers to possible allergies, side effects, reactions, and other complications relevant to each particular patient as that patient is being treated.

Moses Cone Health System in Greensboro, North Carolina, established a 50 percent error reduction as one of three goals for its information infrastructure (the other two are to improve hospital-based clinician productivity by 20 percent and physician productivity by 20 percent). In fact, errors have been reduced by more than two-thirds. Within the first week of going live with a data repository, errors were identified in more than 3 percent of ancillary orders. With automated alerts, this dropped to less than 1 percent. Based on two million annual lab tests, the automated alerts will reduce errors by forty thousand and yield an estimated $1 million in savings annually (Lopez, 1996).

Other health care organizations show similar results. Promedica Health System in Toledo, Ohio, expects to recoup $2 million from its automated alerting function in 1998 and $3 million to $4 million in 1999 (Schneider, 1997). Brigham and Women's Hospital in Boston calculates a $2 million return on investment annually solely from savings in drug costs and the prevention of adverse drug events (Schneider, 1996b, 1996c).

Information technology not only improves efficiencies directly through benefits such as those described above, it also does so indirectly by reducing malpractice liability. The quality of documentation and abundance of missing, incomplete, or poor documentation account for the majority of malpractice losses (Sullivan, 1996). As those in the legal field have noted, paper charting naturally leads to these problems by limiting data entry to either handwriting or dictation and transcription. A recent survey of research by Arthur D. Little (Renner, 1996) showed that 20 percent of paper records had items from another patient's chart, paper charts were missing in 6 percent to 18 percent of patient visits, and information deemed necessary by clinicians was missing 18 to 20 percent of the time, requiring repeat tests or consults for 3 to 5 percent of patients.

Appropriate information technology reduces the liability exposure of a health care organization by reducing errors, improving documentation, providing closed-loop procedure tracking (which prevents a record from being closed before all follow-up actions have been completed), and increasing control over access to confidential information.

Increasing Intelligence and Capacity

Information technology also supports agility by enabling humans to focus on areas in which human capacity may be leveraged to greatest effect. In both medical training and practice, humans have been used to absorb massive amounts of information and perform routine tasks that might better be done in partnership with information systems. Agile organizations increasingly will team computers with providers to maximize both efficiency and effectiveness.

Early evidence suggests that combined human and computer performance exceeds what either can do alone. Radiologists' detection of early lung nodules, for example, is improved with the aid of computers that detect potential nodules and highlight them on the radiograph. Figure 7.1 shows the results of a recent test by Kobayashi and others (1996) comparing the performance of sixteen radiologists reading 120 radiographs with and without computer-aided diagnosis (CAD). The increased performance achieved with CAD is particularly important given the fact that early lung nodules are not detected in 20 to 30 percent of actual positive cases. Similarly, neural networks that use radiologist-extracted features of breast lesions are better able to distinguish between those that are benign and those that are malignant than either attending or radiology residents are able to distinguish working on their own, without computers.

Increasingly, information systems will be used to analyze patterns, make calculations, guide precision treatments, monitor body systems continuously, alert providers to problems, and carry out tasks that would not be feasible or practical otherwise. Some information

Figure 7.1. Radiologists' Reading of Radiographs With and Without CAD

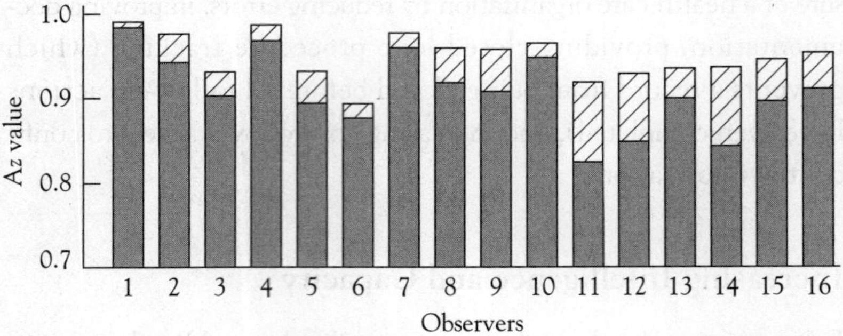

Note: Gray shading represents the Az (azimuth) values for conventional radiograph only. Diagonal stripes correspond to the increase in Az values from using the CAD scheme.

Source: Kobayashi and others (1996).

technologies, such as neural nets, will also be used to minimize error and serve as a second reader in diagnostic tests. PAPNET, for example, does exactly this for Pap smears. Nationally, approximately 20 to 40 percent of smears containing cancerous or precancerous cells are classified as normal. Neural networks reduce this percentage by highlighting the most abnormal-appearing cells for a second review by a cytologist. In a multisite clinical study submitted to the Food and Drug Administration, it was shown that PAPNET detected an additional 30 percent of potentially abnormal cases (Schneider, 1996c, pp. 69–70). Genetic algorithms and neural nets are two powerful new software tools for increasing computer-enhanced intelligence. Technologies such as these will augment but not displace human intelligence and capacity. Those individuals and organizations who know how to combine the two most effectively will reach the highest levels of performance and market agility.

Genetic Algorithms

A genetic algorithm is a computational optimization process that is analogous to biological evolution through natural selection. In biological evolution, fitness is determined by the ability of an animal, for example, a finch or a newt, to attract a mate or obtain food. Analogously, in a system that uses a genetic algorithm such as a critical pathway analyzer, the right balance of treatment and cost savings is determined by finding the optimal outcomes of historical practices.

The genetic algorithm is applied to an ensemble of individuals, each made up of a set of parameters that are candidates for solving the optimization problem. The genetic algorithm proceeds by first evaluating the fitness of the individuals in a population. Fitness is a measure of how well a single set of candidate parameters optimizes the function in question. The fittest individuals are then manipulated to simulate crossbreeding within the population. Finally, a few individuals are subject to random mutations.

Each of the three steps has an effect on the fitness of the population analogous to that on a biological population. In the first step, the best solutions are identified. In the second step, the individuals that are most fit share their genetic code. This increases the probability that the fittest parameter subsets will be propagated throughout the population. In the third step, a few individuals are given some unique genetic code, resulting in parameters that explore the genetic possibilities beyond that of the present population.

After taking the three steps, a new generation is formed, and the process is repeated. Mutations help the population to export regions of the parameter space that are genetically far from the present gene pool. However, by selecting the fitter individuals to crossbreed in each generation, the population is increasingly likely to contain the optimal or near-optimal individuals—that is, the one individual or small set of the individuals that contains the set of parameters optimizing the function in question.

Typically, the "genes" of the genetic algorithm are the streams of bits that the computer uses to represent the numbers that quantify the relevant parameters of the system. From two individuals of the population, then, we get two others that may be more or less fit than their parents. As the process progresses, the population as a whole becomes increasingly fit (Goldberg, 1986) because fit individuals share their genetic code more often than unfit individuals do. A genetic algorithm typically converges to the optimal solution after a few hundred generations.

Machine Learning Using Artificial Neural Networks

The artificial neural network consists of nodes or neurons that are connected to their nearest neighbors through variable-strength connections or weights. We can carry the biological analogy further and call these synapses. Like their biological counterparts, artificial neural networks learn from and adapt to a changing environment. They are robust in the same sense as a biologic neural network in that information is not localized but is distributed throughout the network. That is, just as losing seven brain cells does not result in the loss of seven specific bits of information, such as a telephone number, so in the artificial neural network, the malfunction of a neuron (one of the nodes in the network) does not cause the system to fail. Furthermore, an artificial neural network can be trained by example, allowing the network to gain knowledge that cannot be encoded from first principles.

These qualities allow artificial neural networks to perform useful tasks like screening pathology slides for abnormal tissues or reading zip codes from hand-addressed envelopes.

Artificial neural networks are suited for problems characterized by the need for a machine that learns by example, not from an encoded set of rules. For example, a zip code character recognition system is constructed not by formulating a set of rules that describes what all 8s look like, but rather by showing the computer 8s and adjusting the network connections until the computer responds with "eight." Similarly, with a pathology slide screening system, the screening computer is shown normal and abnormal tissue, and the network connections are adjusted until the computer responds appropriately.

Artificial neural networks interpolate very well, but they rarely extrapolate successfully. That is, a zip code character recognition system trained to recognize the digits 1 through 8 with a wide variation in size, angle, and other parameters would not automatically recognize the digit 9. This may seem obvious in this discrete system where the machine responses are either right or wrong. However, the same principle holds for continuous systems such as predicting airport traffic volumes. For example, if the system was not trained with data from the Christmas holiday season, the volumes predicted for December 23 will be incorrect extrapolations of normal volume patterns.

Conclusion

Information technology is a core strategic asset in health care that holds the keys to effective decision making, clinical practice improvement, optimal resource allocations, agile workforces, and process efficiencies. Organizations that master the use of these technologies secure advantages in speed, cost, and effectiveness.

Recognizing this fact, health care executives have increased spending by 30 percent per year in the past two years. Investments in future years are likely to increase at an even greater rate. Early financial returns and quality gains from these investments have been achieved in a variety of health systems. Ultimately the returns will be measured by a larger transformation as patients manage conditions more effectively from their homes, clinicians and computers partner to diagnose and monitor conditions, providers learn continuously in the context of actual practice, and health systems integrate data to enable greater knowledge. Organizations will "think," work, and communicate in new ways. They will achieve unprecedented agility.

8

Creating the Doctor of Tomorrow

Agility in Medical Education

Morton D. Sosland, David B. Nash

Physicians have to change the way they practice medicine, and medical schools have to change the way they train physicians. Creating the doctor of tomorrow requires a new approach to medical education, one rooted in the new realities of effective medical practice. The agility model offers such an approach.

Environmental Characteristics

The environment in which medical schools must function today shares many of the characteristics of the commercial business environment to which agility was a response: shrinking product lifetimes, simultaneous cooperation and competition, reorganization frenzy, mass customization and market fragmentation, and social values pressures.

Shrinking Product Lifetimes

Like manufacturers, physicians find themselves serving markets characterized by shrinking product lifetimes. For physicians, the "products" they sell are their applications to individual patients of the medical knowledge they possess and the technologies at their disposal. At a time when the clockspeed of medical knowledge change is already unprecedented and still accelerating, the lifetime of any given knowledge-and-technology application is constantly shrinking. To provide the best possible care, that is, to provide *competitive* care, physicians must constantly update their knowledge of which therapies are most appropriate and most effective. If a physician is not doing this, not only are their patients suffering, but the physician is vulnerable to competition from physicians who possess current knowledge and can use the latest technologies. The response of the medical school cannot be *only* to teach well the current state of the health care art. It must do this so that its students will be able to function effectively when they graduate and for the near term after graduation, but it must also train students who expect constant intensive reeducation throughout their professional lives, and it must provide this reeducation.

Cooperation and Competition

Like industrial corporations, medical schools find themselves in a market characterized by simultaneous cooperation and competition among organizations that used to be competitors only. This may take the form of simultaneous competition and cooperation among medical schools for students, or among medical schools, hospitals, and managed care organizations for funding of operations, or among medical schools, hospitals, and government agencies or pharmaceutical companies for research projects.

Reorganization Frenzy

The reorganization frenzy that has afflicted industry for over a decade is also being experienced by the health care sector. Hospitals and medical schools are affiliating and merging. Single hospitals are forming alliances that themselves grow into regional and even national networks. A hospital or practice with minimal managed care involvement today may be part of a managed care network tomorrow. Individual and group provider practices are being merged into hospital alliances and managed care networks at a dizzying pace. There are signs that medical schools, in pursuit of economies of scope as well as of scale, and in anticipation of a heralded oversupply of practitioners, are looking to mergers and networks as models for their own futures.

Customizing for Niche Markets

Not surprisingly, the information technologies that are enabling industry to move from mass production for mass markets to mass customization targeting smaller and smaller niche markets are also enabling health care organizations to treat masses of patients with unprecedented individuality. Using computerized patient records to support a population-based medical care philosophy, physicians can identify individual patients with similar care profiles who are distributed in large population groups or are physically dispersed. These patients can then be offered effective, focused care over their whole lives and in changing care settings. The economies derived from scale no longer require that patients be physically co-located in order to be offered higher-quality and more cost-effective treatment, or preventative care targeting their specific medical conditions, health needs, and the characteristics of their neighborhoods.

Information technology is also enabling increasingly sophisticated global networks of medical researchers, databases, and clinical knowledge. By using the Internet, the World Wide Web, and teleconferencing, medical schools around the world are sharing knowledge and training resources. In the process, medical education is expanding far beyond the traditional campus and classroom.

Social Pressures

There is an increasing recognition today in health care organizations that like a growing number of industrial corporations, they too must internalize prevailing social values. Medical schools are requiring students to become involved in community health programs. An increased focus on clinical outcomes, costs, and efficiency is also being driven by market and societal pressures. The federal government is pressuring medical schools to produce more primary care physicians and fewer specialists. The federal Health Care Financing Administration in 1997 began paying New York State hospitals to reduce their residency positions, and a consensus is emerging that all medical students should have some generalist training, a viewpoint adopted by the Association of American Medical Colleges' Advisory Panel on the Mission and Organization of Medical Schools, established in 1994 "to counsel the association and its constituents on how medical schools can best address their societal missions in the midst of the wrenching changes occurring in the health care system."

What Does Agility Offer?

For a commercial enterprise, to be agile is to be capable of operating profitably in a competitive environment of continually, and unpredictably, changing customer opportunities. A medical school also needs to operate profitably in a similar environment, and thus it too needs to be agile. For a medical school, agility includes the requirement that its "products"—the new physicians it trains—receive the kind of training that will enable them to thrive in *their* agile marketplaces. That is, it is not enough for the medical school to become an agile organization. It must produce physicians who are agile: capable of contributing to the bottom line of a hospital, group practice, or managed care organization that is constantly reorganizing its human and technological resources in response to unpredictably changing marketplace demands and opportunities.

It is more than just an interesting exercise to point out the similarities between the commercial business environment and the environment that medical schools find themselves in. The objective is to gain valuable new insights into how medical schools can respond effectively to the challenges confronting them, challenges that increasingly resemble those confronting businesses. Borrowing from the agile business model, an agile medical school would do the following:

- Bring health care solutions to market that are variable combinations of technology, information, services, and people
- Create highly variable and individualized services that involve their customers in their design

- Leverage the impact of the skills and knowledge of its workforce
- Continually upgrade services and options based on improved technologies and patient and physician preferences
- Develop integrated, continuing relationships among health care professionals, corporations, and empowered health partners that result in lifelong holistic collaborations that improve the health status of entire communities
- Cooperate intensively with other health care partners, including competitors
- Adopt the organizational structure that best serves the customer
- Shift its culture from a command-and-control management philosophy to a "think like an owner" workforce philosophy
- Manage relationships differently: relationships with customers, suppliers, vendors, patients, physicians, employers, and payers
- Create virtual enterprises to sell solutions
- Develop informational networks that cross organizational boundaries
- Develop services built on customer-perceived value and market them successfully

A Market-Pulled Approach

One of the basic concepts underlying agility is responsiveness to markets. Some medical educators are beginning to take a market-oriented approach to changing medical education. Rather than continuing to train medical students and residents the way that they are being trained—ways that reflect early and mid-twentieth-century health care market forces—these educators are suggesting that medical education needs to reflect the distinctive values of today's health care markets. In his president's address at the Association of American Medical Colleges annual meeting in November 1995, Jordan J. Cohen said:

> Academic medicine is an industry. I know we don't like to think of ourselves that way, but stripped to the core, that's clearly what we are and we shouldn't be ashamed to say so. The image of an industry as a grimy, mindless, clanking of machinery, grinding out indistinguishable widgets, is a myopic and outmoded caricature. The reality is that successful industries make things and provide services that people want and need. People want and need well-educated and highly trained physicians, new medical knowledge, and high-quality medical care. That's what our industry makes!
>
> But no industry, however successful, can expect to go on doing business the same way indefinitely. The desires of people change. Their needs change. The world changes. Successful industries change to meet—and to create—new expectations and new realities. And, like it or not, our customers are beginning to express many new expectations and to raise troubling questions about each one of our products—education, research, and clinical services. Are we training the right number and kinds of physicians? Why does our education cost so much? Do we need to re-balance our research agenda with more emphasis on getting products to market faster and doing a more effective job taking care of people with the knowledge we already have? Why are the prices of our health care services so high?

> We are being challenged now to drive our industry—and its production line—into better alignment with the changing needs and expectations of our customers: our students, our patients, the public. [Cohen, 1996]

Elliott and others (1996) have attempted to frame medical education in business terms and respond to the market. They proposed that physician training be viewed in terms of a business model. The assessment of the quality of a residency program, for example, must take into account the values, demands, and requirements of the program's various customers: the trainees themselves, patients, funding agencies, health care employers, medical schools and teaching hospitals, and professional organizations. Are the diverse needs of these customers being met? Medical school education and residency training continues to be based on the view that "doctors know best what it takes to train new doctors":

> This view does not entirely miss the mark—certainly physicians know a great deal about training needs—but it leads to a narrow view of quality. How can a broader view of quality be developed, one that is more responsive to the needs of all those who have stakes in medical education? . . . Quality, as it is understood in many businesses today, begins with a consideration of the people who receive the organization's "products." . . . As applied to residency training, the definition becomes: quality in residency training means meeting or exceeding the needs and reasonable expectations of the residency's customers. [Wartman, 1994]

Who are these customers and what are their needs?

The trainees' needs include the expectation that "they will be selected fairly, receive training sufficient to meet their future needs, receive fair compensation, receive fair assessment of their skills, and have at the end of their training adequate opportunities to practice in personally rewarding settings" (Elliott and others, 1996, p. 245).

The patients and their families "want competent, compassionate, culturally sensitive, and cost-effective care" (Elliott and others, 1996, p. 245). They also need an adequate number of physicians, especially in underserved areas. The funding agencies expect that other customers' needs will be satisfied, such as the patients'. They also demand cost-effective training that meets the needs of specific areas and underserved populations.

The health care payer, for example, managed care organizations, "expect training programs to produce practitioners who understand third-party payer concerns, practice within established utilization-management guidelines, are focused on customer needs and concerns, and understand the flexible nature of physicians' roles and responsibilities" (Elliott and others, 1996, p. 245). They also expect physicians to be able to work with other health care providers, and to be able to participate in administrative activities such as utilization review and quality improvement.

Training centers such as medical schools and teaching hospitals expect residency programs to help them develop practitioners, professional leaders, researchers, and educators.

Finally, professional organizations, such as the American Medical Association, "need ethical, competent practitioners to represent, promote, and advance their professions" (Elliott and others, 1996, p. 245).

The Current Need for Agility

Managed care companies, which insure as many as 130 million people in this country, have changed the focus of health care and in the process placed new demands on physicians. In a 1996 editorial in the *Journal of the American Medical Association*, David Blumenthal and Samuel O. Thier wrote:

> Compared with physicians in traditional fee-for-service practice, physicians practicing in managed care settings provide more ambulatory care and less inpatient care, face new pressures to practice cost-effectively and to work in interdisciplinary teams, must deal with new forms of payment and administrative controls, and are required to think about maintaining the health of populations rather than just individual patients.
>
> Today's physicians require a new set of skills and knowledge to work effectively in this new environment. The question is where are they going to get these skills and knowledge? Are medical schools providing it or do physicians have to pick it up after their residencies in on-the-job training? Some would argue that medical schools and residency programs have until now not been providing their graduates with the requisite skills that the market is demanding. [p. 726]

Another author writes that managers of health maintenance organizations (HMOs) estimate it takes one to two years of additional experience (over traditional training) to prepare graduates of U.S. residencies for practice in a managed care environment (Shine, 1996). Some medical schools and residency programs have in fact begun adding courses on managed care and clinical experiences in managed care environments, but the response has been slow. According to an article that appeared in *JAMA* in September 1996, most medical schools are not requiring their students to gain experience working in managed care settings (Veloski and others, 1996).

In 1995 and 1996, an average of only 16 percent of schools required all of their students to have clerkships or other clinical experiences in a group or staff model HMO. In 46 percent of schools, some students spent some time in an HMO during their clerkships or introduction to clinical medicine and physical diagnosis courses. Although less than half of medical schools had students working in

HMOs, about 85 percent of schools may have been at least exposing students to managed care through required clinical experiences in ambulatory, community-based settings (Veloski and others, 1996).

Veloski and others (1996) note that even medical schools that do have rotations in managed care settings are for the most part using these settings in the same way they are using other outpatient settings: to teach clinical skills. They are not focusing on such skills as cost-effective care or quality management, skills their students will be expected to possess when they work in managed care settings.

The need is clear for medical schools to do a better job of matching medical education to the distinctive requirements of the health care environment as it is now, not as it used to be.

The Agile Response

Change in medical education comes slowly, but there are a number of promising developments to point to, especially in response to the requirements of practicing medicine in managed care settings.

The Partnerships for Quality Education (PQE) program was started in 1996 by the Pew Charitable Trusts to create educational partnerships between medical schools and managed care companies. This represents an agile response in that medical schools are now cooperating with managed care companies to improve the way they train students. Consistent with the agility model, managed care companies can be viewed by medical schools as customers (for new physicians) or as competitors for health care dollars. As customers, the agile response is to work with them in spite of the fact that they are concurrently competitors to provide them with win-win solutions to their problems rather than take-it-or-leave-it products. Jefferson Medical College, for example, has introduced courses on managed care and provides a fellowship sponsored by a managed care company.

Information technology is enabling medical training that is continually updated with the latest knowledge using computer databases. Information networks are allowing medical education to cross organizational boundaries with the goal, already in part realized, of developing a virtual university. There is increased emphasis on developing services and educating medical students and residents based on what the customer (the public) wants. This includes increased student involvement in community projects, often in underserved areas.

Medical schools have begun to offer courses, and in at least one case a residency program, on complementary (alternative) medicine. This move is symptomatic of an acceptance of customer-perceived value—reflected in the growing proportion of health care dollars that the public is spending on alternative therapies—as a driver of curriculum reform.

Partnerships for Quality Education

Funded by the Pew Charitable Trusts in a grant to Harvard Pilgrim Health Care in the amount of $8.3 million over a three-year period, PQE is an example of how leading academic health centers and managed care organizations can collaborate to train medical students, residents, and practicing physicians to provide high-quality managed patient care. For the academic health center, collaboration with managed care organizations fulfills "the need for outpatient training sites and their responsibility to ensure that their residents—and faculty—are adequately trained in managed care skills." Concurrently, the managed care organization gains "preferred access to research results and academic resources in areas such as ethics and epidemiology; the marketing advantage that can come from association with an academic institution; the opportunity to use residents to test strategies for changing physician behavior; the ability to use teaching programs to attract physicians to areas in which the MCO needs physicians; and the advantages of having a partnership with one of their major tertiary providers" (March and Moore, 1997, p. 182).

Furthermore, academic health centers, which have "traditionally held a special place in society," are "increasingly under fire for high costs, overproduction of specialists and lack of commitment to local communities" (March and Moore, 1997, p. 182). Managed care organizations, in turn, are suffering an erosion of public confidence because their financial models are perceived to drive care provision criteria. Through PQE, each helps the other increase confidence that they are serving the public well in their respective ways.

These are the goals of PQE:

- To determine how partnerships can be good for business and good for education
- To highlight the benefits of academic partnerships for the public and for the purchasers of health care
- To support established partnerships and help those considering new alliances
- To develop innovative models for medical education that can be replicated by partnerships across the country
- To initiate advancements in primary care medical education

By partnering with managed care organizations, academic health centers can do the following:

- Ensure that residents are prepared to practice comfortably and effectively in managed care environments
- Give residents the skills to interact with managed care organizations to ensure high-quality patient care
- Train medical students in managed care concepts and practices

- Provide residents with an insider's view of how managed care organizations work

Academic partnerships allow managed care organizations to do the following:

- Shape medical education to meet their needs better
- Take a leadership role in medical education
- Position themselves as a quality provider in the marketplace by advertising, "If you want a good doctor, find one who teaches"
- Recruit better-trained physicians
- Minimize the cost of retraining physicians in the skills and competencies of managed care
- Develop research relationships that have beneficial bottom-line effects

PQE encompasses seven primary projects, ranging from faculty development to managed Medicaid.

The Tufts Managed Care Institute: Faculty Development

The Tufts Managed Care Institute (TMCI) was formed in 1995 by Tufts University School of Medicine and Tufts Health Plan, a Massachusetts-based independent practice association network model HMO. Through PQE, TMCI is developing a managed care curriculum for primary care residents. This is a joint effort of the medical school, health plan, internal medicine, and family medicine residency training programs at two affiliated hospitals and physicians from two local community practices.

The curriculum includes an introduction to managed care, patient-centered care, ambulatory practice guidelines, and a managed care rotation in a four-week block that combines clinical practice with activities and projects related to managed care topics. The managed care topics contain a historical and economic component, the basics of utilization management, an introduction to capitation, quality assessment in the prepaid practice, and ethical issues.

The program is developing teaching modules that can be exported to other sites. This includes an interactive CD-ROM on managed care called *The Digital Preceptor*, which will have clinical cases that teach managed care principles. In the future, *The Digital Preceptor* may be made available on-line when Internet graphics and video are strong enough to support it.

Hands-on managed care experience will take place in local community practices and in the residency programs. For example, at Newton-Wellesley Hospital, medical residents are being given experience with clinical practice guidelines utilizing evidence-based medicine. Residents will be asked to do chart audits of their own and of their colleagues' practice patterns to assess the use of practice guidelines.

At Beverly Hospital, the residency directors are developing a program on patient-centered care from a managed care perspective. They will work on communication skills, involving patients and their families in clinical decisions, and ethical issues. These skills will be studied in the context of patient and population perspectives as well as cost and quality issues.

One department chief and residency program director of an affiliated hospital reported that the TMCI already "has changed the way I teach. Last night our residents admitted a woman in a diabetic coma. This morning I asked them, 'If you were the head of a large HMO responsible for the health of a population, what would you do to prevent this from happening again?'"

Beyond PQE, TMCI is involved in a host of other activities to integrate managed care topics into medical education. The goal of TMCI at its inception was to help "produce a new generation of medical practitioners whose understanding of their own responsibility goes beyond practicing good medical care to practicing the best, most cost-effective medicine, recognizing their responsibility for the quality and cost of care" (Phillips, Lee, Berman, and Madoff, 1997, p. 349). In pursuit of this goal, TMCI is developing educational programs for practicing health care professionals and for medical students and residents. These programs integrate managed care principles and practices into medical school cases, courses, and clerkships. Training is also offered to faculty through workshops and through increased communication with managed care executives.

The medical student curriculum covers six subjects:

- *Historical and economic overview of managed care*. This material encompasses financing and health care delivery systems, ranging from traditional fee for service to managed care. The importance of risk-sharing arrangements is covered as it affects the roles and responsibilities of providers, patients, and payers.

- *Coordination, collaboration, and communication*. As managed care requires efficient resource utilization, there is an increased need for communication and collaboration among physicians, other health care practitioners, patients, and managed care plans.

- *Efficient clinical care*. This includes efficient care processes and evidence-based clinical decision making, utilization and resource management, health promotion, disease prevention, and ethical analysis.

- *Quality assessment and improvement*. This covers continuous improvement approaches and tools, as well as assessment of quality, outcomes, health status, patient satisfaction, and physician satisfaction.

- *Working with managed care plans*. Students become familiar with financing and risk arrangements. They learn to analyze a health plan's mission, goals, structure, and functions and how to communicate with health plans and purchasers.

- *Medical practice management*. Students learn about utilization criteria and financial information systems, as well as skills for working with professional and support staff, and how to set up scheduling and telephone systems to improve patient access.

In implementing its programs, TMCI has concentrated on curriculum integration, faculty involvement and development, participation of managed care faculty, experiential learning, and teamwork and collaboration. The objective is to blend managed care into the existing curriculum—into the classes, problem-based learning cases, and clerkships—as opposed to creating stand-alone managed care courses. In addition, a managed care criterion has been incorporated into the evaluations of third-year students in their clinical rotations, including attention to cost and efficiency issues in diagnosis and treatment.

Georgetown University–Kaiser Permanente: Managed Care Ethics

For their PQE project, Georgetown University School of Medicine and Kaiser Permanente are focusing on ethical issues distinctive of managed care and the development of tools to measure ethical attitudes. Three activities are being funded through PQE. One is the development of a Kaiser-owned site in a family-centered practice in downtown Washington, D.C., into a model for all internal medicine and pediatrics residents receiving outpatient training. The site will include several examination rooms with videotaping capabilities so that students can practice and review patient encounters, such as obtaining advance directives from patients. The residents will be trained in using the computer network–based Kaiser Patient Information System, which allows them to review lab results, receive messages, e-mail the clinic nurse for callbacks, and access the Internet and reference material. A number of residents will be using an advanced voice-activated medical record system.

A second activity uses this same practice model to develop a managed care ethics curriculum taught by faculty from Kaiser and the Georgetown Center for Clinical Bioethics. In addition to integrating the ethics component into clinical cases and lectures, each resident will work on a project with a mentor in quality and ethics and also be required to serve on the Kaiser Ethics Committee.

The third activity also uses the practice model, this time to develop a curriculum in quality management and quality improvement.

Kaiser views the partnership with Georgetown as a prototype that it plans to use throughout the Kaiser system. As with the other PQE projects, the plan is to expand its application by sharing its results and techniques with other academic health centers and other managed care organizations.

Legacy Health System and Regence Blue Cross: Teaching

Legacy Health System and Regence Blue Cross–Blue Shield in Oregon are working with the HealthFirst Medical Group, which runs a number of clinics, and with Mulliken Emanuel, an internal medicine practice, to develop new teaching materials. They are collaborating on a number of projects, including development of a work group on ethical issues related to managed care, quality improvement projects, and residency training. Although this program does not involve a specific medical school, one of its components is to implement a residency program.

As part of the PQE project, the partnership plans to develop and implement a managed care curriculum, develop two additional for-profit community sites for teaching at group practice sites, and take the lead in disseminating the partnership model throughout the Blue Cross–Blue Shield network.

The program's goal is to prepare residents better to work in a managed care environment. The program will include seminars in health policy, quality improvement, prevention and health risk appraisal, and chronic disease management and geriatrics. Residents will also work on projects related to managed care.

The Continuous Quality Improvement (CQI) curriculum will help residents to understand the entire process used by a managed care organization, not strictly the one-on-one patient encounter. CQI will be applied to residency training by developing strategies to treat common diagnoses focusing on using systemwide resources available to patients and providers. Each month, residents at different sites will compare how they responded to common diagnoses and then work on process improvements that can benefit the whole system. Regence Blue Cross–Blue Shield of Oregon will provide coaches to assist in teaching this form of process improvement.

Through an initiative sponsored by the American Geriatrics Society, geriatrics training is being added to the program as part of an effort to provide a continuum of care—what in agility terms is an individualized customer solution rather than a stand-alone service or product. The plan is to develop citywide educational sessions in different disciplines to provide a multidisciplinary approach to geriatric care.

In parallel with its PQE project, Legacy Health System is working with the Robert Wood Johnson Foundation to study health risk appraisals and intervention in the geriatric population. Medical residents participating in the PQE program would be able to work on this project to learn about patient assessment and effective use of community resources. They will learn firsthand about the common practice of profiling as they will receive feedback regarding their financial performance as staff physicians would. This approach to teaching residents about managed care will be evaluated by measuring patient, resident, and preceptor satisfaction. The residents will also be involved in a quality improvement project on the program itself.

Harvard Pilgrim–Harvard Medical: Research Partnerships

Harvard Pilgrim Health Care and Harvard Medical School are studying the creation of joint academic health center–managed care organization clinical research networks. In June 1996, Pew Charitable Trusts awarded $8.3 million to Harvard Pilgrim Health Care to undertake a national initiative to increase the number of educational partnerships between academic health centers and managed care organizations. Harvard Pilgrim has been collaborating with Harvard Medical School in teaching and research for the past twenty-five years. In 1991, they formalized this partnership when they formed the joint Department of Ambulatory Care and Prevention.

Under their PQE grant, they have undertaken five initiatives:

- Design and pilot a faculty development program.
- Develop and implement a managed care curriculum for third-year medical students. Managed care topics have been integrated into a new year-long longitudinal primary care clerkship along the following themes: advanced communication, time-efficient medical interviewing, evidence-based medicine, practice analysis, and clinical quality improvement. Forty of the 150 students are assigned to Harvard Pilgrim Health Care sites.
- Design and implement a clinical research network.
- Develop a program to train residents to analyze and shape the practices in which they work.
- Analyze the partnership and develop recommendations for strengthening it and exporting it to the other seven participating organizations.

Ford–Case Western Reserve: Financing for Graduate Medical Education

The PQE partnership of Henry Ford Health System and Case Western Reserve University School of Medicine is developing and implementing an alternative payment model for graduate medical education. Included in this topic is the issue of how to improve the incentives for individual teaching faculty and the clinic sites where teaching occurs. They are focusing in particular on the costs of ambulatory teaching and methods for proper compensation because more and more teaching will be done in ambulatory settings. The partnership is also developing an innovative model residency training site. The model builds on the community-oriented primary care programs of the late 1960s by integrating managed care, quality improvement, and evidence-based medicine into the curriculum. Residents will use the training site to learn and practice these skills.

As part of clinical process improvement at this site, population surveying is being done. Screening instruments were reviewed by the faculty in an attempt to begin the process of population stratification. They looked at several instruments including a biomedically based health quiz and others that are more socially and community based. In addition, outcome measures are being identified that cover clinical, functional, satisfaction, and cost outcomes. These outcome measures will be incorporated into the clinical information system used by physicians and residents.

Cornell/Empire and Penn/Independence: Feedback Systems for Resident Practices

The partnerships of Cornell University Medical College with New York Hospital and Empire Blue Cross–Blue Shield and of the University of Pennsylvania with Independence Blue Cross are working on feedback systems to assess how residents are performing from a payer's as well as from a provider's perspective. The program integrates medical residency training with a rotation in a managed care setting. The two- or four-week rotation educates residents in health care economics, policy, quality, and the principles of managed care. The program fosters the use of quality practice measures as tools to improve the delivery of care.

Residents in the Cornell–New York Hospital program rotate through a number of Empire's departments, including utilization management, quality, legal, pharmacy, medical policy, strategic planning, fraud and abuse, financial, and actuarial. They participate in operational activities at Empire: committee meetings, operations, claims processing, customer service, and quality improvement efforts. When asked to share opinions of the program in a survey, one resident wrote, "I was very impressed by the efforts of Empire to ensure quality in health care . . . my views of managed care have shifted somewhat from 'managed cost' to improving quality while decreasing costs." The program includes a physician practice profiling system to teach residents how to evaluate their own practices and how to engage in CQI. Plans call for a study to be conducted on patient satisfaction with care.

Concurrently, data on five thousand patients seen by forty second-year residents over a nine-month period are being collected. The data will be used to measure clinical outcomes among the different residents, focusing initially on the management of diabetes, hypertension, and depression. In addition, Empire is providing claims data to residents for research projects to identify patterns and trends on quality of care, resource utilization, and patient satisfaction. One resident conducted a study entitled "Defining the Intrinsic Systemic Barriers to Effective Health Care Delivery: Observations from Latinos at an Academic Outpatient Center." The resident put together a focus group to identify the needs of a defined patient population and used managed care data to measure access to care.

The University of Pennsylvania Health System and Independence Blue Cross partnership is developing a quality measurement and feedback system for use with primary care resident practices. This partnership began as a direct result of the PQE program and involves two activities: (1) a three-week administrative block rotation at Independence Blue Cross for primary care residents and (2) implementation of a system for monitoring resident practices in the areas of prevention, utilization, disease management, and patient satisfaction. Plans are in place to create report cards for residents, which will include individual and group quality data.

UNM-Lovelace: Managed Medicaid

The University of New Mexico School of Medicine and Lovelace Health System are exploring a new risk-sharing relationship through the PQE program. Their grant is for developing a partnership practice to share the care of between four thousand and five thousand managed Medicaid patients in a resident-faculty setting. They will also develop a curriculum and training methods for the residents so they can be integrated into the care of these patients cost-effectively. Finally, as with the other PQE projects, this is being developed so that it can be packaged for use by other academic health center–managed care organization partnerships.

A Lovelace physician will be assigned to the clinic to teach faculty and residents. Topics to be covered will include managed care principles, population-based medicine, quality management, cost and utilization management, disease management approaches, the importance of practice profiling and data feedback, ethical issues, referral issues, patient satisfaction, and team decision making. The curriculum will be taught through a mix of didactic sessions, multidisciplinary problem-based tutorials, hands-on experience with selected patients, and rotations. Teaching the medical school faculty is seen as a critical component of the program so they will be able to serve as managed care preceptors for their residents.

Information systems will be installed to support the managed care practice and for quality improvement. Residents will use the information systems to gain experience in these processes and in data feedback. A variety of utilization and clinical data feedback measures and practice profiling reports will be used to prepare the residents for work in a managed care setting.

Jefferson Medical College: An Agile Response

Although Jefferson Medical College is not a direct participant in the PQE, one of us (DBN) is the associate director of the PQE program. Jefferson is responding with agility to the changes in its markets in a number of ways. First-year medical students are required to take a two-and-a-half week course, Health Policy: An Introduction to the Health Care System, that covers the cost of health care, the health insurance system, paying the hospital and paying the physician, quality and outcomes, physician responsibility for quality, practice guidelines, information and data resources, Total Quality Management, physician/hospital/HMO report cards, future practice alternatives, and the future of the health care system.

Second-year medical students take a seminar entitled, Is Big Brother Watching You? What Is Quality and How Do You Measure It? The course description reads: "While cost containment for health care was the hallmark of the 1980s, providing value—high quality at reasonable cost—will be the theme for the 1990s. Learn how you will be evaluated once you are a practicing physician."

A senior elective is also offered in health policy that reflects on all of these issues in more detail.

In an example of cooperation with other health care partners, Jefferson has had an Aetna–U.S. Healthcare Fellowship Program that supported two postresidency physicians with one-year fellowships. The curriculum covered such topics as biostatistics and epidemiology, medical informatics, theory and practice of managed care, managed care finance, integrated health care systems, quality assessment and improvement, clinical parameters and guidelines, utilization management, and risk management. The fellowship, which is funded primarily by Aetna–U.S. Healthcare, has as its mission to train physicians to understand the theory and practice of quality management. Graduates of the program are currently working in leadership positions in national managed health care firms.

Another program at Jefferson that reflects an agile response to the demands of some students and to the demands of the market is the combined five-year M.D./M.B.A. program with Widener College. The management training and M.B.A. are particularly useful for physicians who are seeking to work as executives in managed care firms, hospitals, or other health care companies.

Information Technology

A different kind of agile response by medical schools involves the use of information technology in medical education. The goals of the project are to use information technology to teach basic sciences, reach distant learners, improve the connection with alumni and other affiliated health care providers, and improve collaboration between Jefferson and non-Jefferson researchers.

The combined use of telecommunications and computer technologies has enabled Jefferson to redefine its educational market. The vision, which is already in part a reality, is to create a "virtual university" using Jefferson's World Wide Web system. It is a new learning environment that people outside of Jefferson can access whether they are in Philadelphia or anywhere else. The system, known as JEFFLINE, is a World Wide Web–based knowledge and education system. Meeting the need for improving knowledge management skills among Jefferson medical students and residents, it is also available to students from other universities that have agreements with Jefferson. The system can be accessed by health care providers within the Jefferson health system, as well as Jefferson alumni. The evolving virtual university allows for independent learning and is seen as part of the trend from teaching in "wet labs" to computer simulation.

Jefferson's Hypermedia TJU Electronic Curriculum (HyTEC), now in development, will permit students to take courses on the computer whenever or wherever they want. Students will have access to electronic databases of text and images, electronic books and journals, independent learning modules, live class sessions, e-mail and bulletin boards, and faculty mentors and other collaborators. A number of global projects are already tied into Jefferson's virtual university. The Ultrasound Research and Education Institute, for example, links Jefferson's Division of Diagnostic Ultrasound with health care facilities around the world, among them the Heim Pal Children's Hospital in Hungary.

Jefferson is working with three partners in Romania through the U.S. Agency for International Development and the American International Health Alliance to assist Romania in its efforts to reduce environmental and occupational health problems in the region of Transylvania. The three Romanian partners—the Center for Medical Research, the Sanitary Police, and the Hospital for Occupational Disease—are located in Cluj-Napoca, the capital of Transylvania. Focusing on informatics, pulmonary medicine, and occupational and environmental health, the partnership has these goals:

- Improving access to information and communication in a way that meets the unique needs of the Romanian partners
- Developing techniques for gathering, manipulating, using, and sharing research data
- Developing models for intervention for two major health care problems: pulmonary disease and exposure to toxic solvents and safeguarding the health of health care workers
- Introducing new programs that should have a major impact on health care: encouraging aftercare and case management with an emphasis on rehabilitation, and encouraging smoke-free environments and smoking cessation
- Providing specialized training for health care workers, especially those in areas related to occupational and environmental medicine

Jefferson has begun work on what it calls the Learning Infrastructure Project, whose mission is "to create new learning environments that harness the power of information technology and instructional design principles to improve the quality of teaching and learning, contain or reduce rising costs, and provide greater access to the resources of Thomas Jefferson University for collaborative research." The project is an agile response to a number of local and global trends:

- The need for knowledge management skills
- The need for independent learning, especially computer-based learning
- Growing demand for problem-based learning
- The shift from teaching in wet labs to computer simulations
- The shift from teaching clinical skills in hospital to teaching in an ambulatory care setting
- Rapidly expanding national and international computer networking
- The need to retrain health professionals to serve as generalists
- Alumni desire to stay connected to Thomas Jefferson University
- The need for Jefferson to have a greater international presence
- The fact that 75 percent of the workforce will need retraining by the year 2000, according to the American Society for Training and Development

Jefferson recognizes that as clinical education continues to move out of the hospital to the ambulatory care setting, information technology can be used to ensure that students still get a high-quality educational experience. By using this technology appropriately, the students can have access to medical databases and faculty mentors from wherever they may be. They can also have access to content specifically developed for each clinical rotation, such as on-line case studies and patient simulations. Faculty can use the information technology to track students' performance on a regular basis. The system can also provide continuous training to residents and affiliated physicians, helping them to keep up with the rapidly changing medical knowledge base.

Community Outreach Programs

Involvement in communities can represent an agile response to prevailing social values. By encouraging medical students to take active roles in helping underserved populations, medical schools are helping to produce future physicians who will be responsive to the needs of society's most vulnerable members. Jefferson has a number of programs in which students can gain medical experience working with the underserved.

Bridging the Gaps is a seven-week paid summer experience in which students in various health professions work in the community in multidisciplinary teams on community health projects designed to improve the quality of life. All of Philadelphia's medical schools currently participate in the program. Since it began in 1991, the program has grown from 20 medical students from one medical school to 148 students from a variety of schools, including social work, law, nursing, dental, and art therapy. Student teams address a range of problems, including homelessness, health literacy, tuberculosis treatment, sickle cell anemia, drug addiction, nutrition, immunization, and maternal and child health. In addition to their work, students receive training on a range of topics: different health belief systems, use of conventional and nontraditional health promotion resources and techniques, comparisons of different types of health insurance systems, and the historical, ideological, and political factors that have shaped American safety net programs.

Another community outreach program is the student-run JeffHOPE clinic (Jefferson Health Opportunities, Prevention, and Education). Through JeffHOPE, students and faculty volunteers run a homeless shelter clinic. Students have also assisted in a number of studies, including one on the prevalence of HIV and tuberculosis among the homeless population. The JeffHOPE program has become multidisciplinary, with the Jefferson College of the Health Professions faculty and students teaching medical students about allied health therapies appropriate for the homeless population.

Alternative Medicine

Until recently, American medical schools have virtually ignored alternative medicine despite its growing popularity among the public. Most medical educators have viewed alternative medicine as untested, unscientific medicine not worthy of being taught in medical schools. Many conventional doctors have labeled it as quackery. These attitudes are now changing as medical schools begin to acknowledge the deep public commitment to alternative medicine.

Eisenberg and others (1993) examined the extent to which the American public uses unconventional therapies, defined as "medical interventions not widely taught at U.S. medical schools or generally available at U.S. hospitals": relaxation techniques, chiropractic, massage, imagery, spiritual healing, commercial weight loss programs, special lifestyle diets, herbal medicine, megavitamin therapy, self-help groups, energy healing, biofeedback, hypnosis, homeopathy, and acupuncture. The study determined that 34 percent of the American public paid $13.7 billion in 1990 for these unconventional treatments. Americans made an estimated 425 million visits to unconventional therapy providers compared to 388 million visits to primary care physicians. A milestone for alternative medicine was reached in 1992 with the formation of the National Institutes of Health Office of Alternative Medicine, a clear recognition that alternative therapies are integral to the American health care system.

What has been the agile response of medical schools? According to the Association of American Medical Colleges, over seventy medical schools currently offer elective courses in alternative medicine or cover the topic in some way in their curriculum. Jefferson Medical College, for example, offers several such courses. Alternative/Complementary Medicine is available to sophomore medical students and covers various philosophies of healing, examines the research evidence supporting their efficacy, and offers strategies for integrating conventional and alternative medicine. Topics include acupuncture, bodywork, herbal medicine, homeopathy, mind-body techniques, nutritional therapies, and spirituality. Stress Management for Medical Students covers mindfulness meditation, breathing techniques, muscle tension release techniques, and cognitive strategies for reducing distraction and anxiety. The course description reads: "This seminar is an excellent introduction to the field of Mind-Body Medicine. Clinical studies have shown beneficial effects of mind-body techniques in treating pain, anxiety, depression, and cardiovascular disease. You will gain first-hand experience with techniques you may wish to prescribe for your future patients."

In July 1997, the University of Arizona College of Medicine began a first-of-its-kind fellowship, one that combines study of conventional and alternative medicine. The Program in Integrative Medicine is a two-year fellowship covering healing-oriented medicine, the art of medicine, research design and evaluation, mind-body medicine, spirituality and medicine, nutritional medicine, phytomedicine, energy medicine, and lifestyle medicine. It was introduced in response to "a growing demand from physicians for a standardized curriculum of training in healing-oriented medicine from an accredited academic institution" (University of Arizona, n.d.).

The program description defines integrative medicine as seeking "to combine the best ideas and practices of conventional and alternative medicine into cost-effective treatments that will be in the best interests of patients and that aim to stimulate the body's natural healing potential" (University of Arizona, n.d.). Its primary therapeutic modalities are guided imagery and hypnotherapy, acupuncture, basic homeopathy, and osteopathic manipulative therapy. In the words of program director Andrew Weil,

> Imagine a future world in which medicine was oriented toward healing rather than disease, where doctors believed in the natural healing capacity of human beings and emphasized prevention above treatment. . . . In such a world doctors and patients would be partners working toward the same ends, with malpractice litigation a rare event rather than commonplace. Insurance companies would happily reimburse for preventive education and natural treatments, knowing these efforts were in their own best interests. [University of Arizona, n.d.]

The Future of Medical Education

A medical school that seeks to thrive in the rapidly changing health care market will respond with agility to meet its demands. Agile medical schools will ride the wave of change, wherever that wave may go. The medical school initiatives described here are harbingers of what all successful medical schools will be doing in the near future.

The medical schools of the early twenty-first century will have close collaborative relationships with the broad public and its values, with the communities they serve, with payers, such as managed care companies, with their medical students, and with a spectrum of health care providers. The more they involve all of these customers in the design of their programs, the more relevant the programs, and the medical schools themselves, will be to the health care market.

Jordan Cohen, president of the American Association of Medical Colleges, stressed in his 1995 presidential address the importance of establishing true school-community partnerships so that "academic medicine would become much better informed about the needs in their regions for various kinds of health care providers, and about the solvable health problems that require attention by investigators and clinicians." He spoke of developing regional medical education consortia that would be responsible "for adjusting the number and distribution of training positions in response to evolving regional needs." These regional consortia would also be responsible for the quality and the educational content of the medical schools and residency programs in their regions.

Nicole Lurie (1996) describes eight domains of knowledge that physicians require in the managed care environment: epidemiologic thinking, human behavior, organizational behavior, information systems, quality measurement and improvement, health care financing and delivery, ethics, and systems-based care. She writes: "Many plans now view their enrollees as 'populations,' and see their role as manager and promoter of the health of these populations. This implies not only managing the health of an individual through the one-on-one doctor-patient encounter, but also the implementation of population-based strategies to improve the health of their enrollees" (p. 1045).

The bottom line is that medical students must acquire a new set of skills that are just now beginning to be taught. Collaborative efforts such as the PQE projects are the kinds of changes that will have to be put in place to ensure that future medical students gain these skills. Medical schools are faced with the challenge of a rapidly changing health care environment; only a structural transformation of the entire health care system, from the education of providers to the cost structure of services, is an acceptable response. Agility is a strategic model that medical schools can embrace in anticipation of what will surely be tomorrow's still-changing health care environment.

9

Creating Agile Health Care Organizations

Carol B. Graham

In the preceding eight chapters, we have reviewed agility theory, cited examples of its application in other industries, looked at some strategies that have been employed successfully in instances of organizational migration to agility, and highlighted specific examples of how agility is being deployed in health care settings. This chapter offers practical assistance for health care professionals who want to use the agility model to help their own organizations achieve bold new goals.

Those wishing to employ the agility model within their own organizations or in collaboration with other organizations will focus on ways to link their core competencies to identify, create, produce, and sustain innovative health care solutions, rather than continuing traditional patterns of episodic acute care. Employing dynamic links among partner organizations to customize sets of core competencies to take advantage of different market opportunities, the agile health care system will anticipate customer trends and needs. Indeed, it may even create those needs through health education and promoting the value that new solutions will have for customers.

Good communication at and between all levels of the new system is vital. Communication extends beyond the need for tools and interfaces that provide seamless information access and exchange. Information management systems are crucial, but the value of communication lies in the ways in which people use the information they receive. Thus, a climate must be created in which not only is it safe to ask and safe to tell, but individual employees, teams, and participating organizations are in fact rewarded on the basis of the contributions that they make to the enhancement of the networks they are part of. Encouraging a network-focused entrepreneurial spirit among employees at all levels of an organization is one of the primary responsibilities of the leadership required to create an agile health care system.

Collaboration: The Common Denominator

If there is a single thread that runs through any implementation of agility in any organization, it surely is collaboration: working cooperatively with the distributed human and physical resources of a single organization, and working with resources distributed across multiple organizations. The former is difficult because of inherited power structures that promote internal competition and fiefdoms, but need and common sense can work wonders. Understanding how to work in a truly cooperative mode with other organizations to produce solutions jointly under the pressures of an agile competitive environment requires out-of-the-box thinking about collaboration.

Although some pioneering work has been done in applying the principles of agility to the development of next-generation health care systems, no clear road map has been drawn. Moreover, no one road map could possibly suffice to direct the migration to agility of all organizations. There is no one right way to organize and operate an agile enterprise. The paths to agility are as diverse as organizations themselves, and no single implementation will ever meet all of the changing needs of health care consumers, providers, and payers.

Furthermore, it is becoming increasingly clear that health care businesses, like their counterparts in other industries, can no longer afford to operate in a strategic vacuum, focused solely on marshaling their internal resources to meet their customers' needs. Quite the contrary. Visionary health care professionals understand that whatever model they develop to compete effectively in the newly commercialized and constantly changing health care environment, collaboration with other organizations (and even with competitors) will be crucial to their success. Thus, although there is no one-size-fits-all agile health care organization, there is one element of agility that will inevitably be common to all implementations: collaborative relationships.

How to put into systematic practice the episodic lessons that people and organizations have learned—from their own experiences, at least, but ideally from those of others—is proving to be an elusive goal. Some models for strategic, enterprise-wide application of agility have been developed and are presented briefly here. They are helpful in demonstrating how health care professionals can begin to identify and leverage useful tactics, while discarding less value-adding ones.

The Interprise Model

In *Cooperate to Compete: Building Agile Business Relationships* (1996) Preiss, Goldman, and Nagel described the "interprise" as the next-generation agile commercial enterprise. Unlike the traditional enterprise, which has well-defined boundaries that set it off from suppliers, customers, partners, and competitors, the interprise has very fuzzy boundaries.

To integrate all of the resources necessary to produce solutions, the agile interprise must link its business, information, and service delivery processes to those of all of the other companies that are stakeholders in the solution creation and marketing process. It thereby achieves speed, acquires access to complementary competencies, and reduces costs—but in the process, it must give up a measure of autonomy and independence. It must learn to share and support the protocols that, for example, allow for electronic commerce and functional interoperability of information systems and production processes.

As an integrated enterprise, an organization's continued well-being becomes dependent on the continuing well-being of the organizations to which it is coupled. Goldman compares the traditional enterprise to a Machiavellian city-state, intensely centered on its own interest, opportunistically exploiting other enterprises to its immediate benefit. In contrast, he compares the interprise to a node in a network of constantly changing but consistently win-win relationships. Preiss, Goldman, and Nagel further characterize the interprise as intensively leveraging knowledge across its extended linkages to design processes that effectively meet the needs of all stakeholders.

An interprise created to maximize the competitiveness of a hospital and its medical staff in capturing new patients would not be content simply to launch a physician referral service and then implement a shared electronic record-keeping system for the hospital and the physicians' offices. Rather, it would begin by asking the stakeholders involved—hospital support as well as professional personnel, management information system vendors, regional employers, HMOs, and insurance carriers—to identify modes of collective operation that would support long-term individual advantage. Certainly it would stress cooperative operational relationships among suppliers, vendors, and payers. And it would create an entrepreneurial environment inside the interprise that encouraged and rewarded every employee to "think like an owner."

The interprise embraces constant change in its marketplace as a positive business factor, a source of new opportunities to create competitive advantage, not a negative condition to be avoided. Its adaptive organizational structure and cross-functional teams allow it to turn on a dime when market change demands it. Its interactive relationships with customers, suppliers, and payers enable it to provide a continually expanding array of solutions to meet the needs of individual customers. And above all, the interprise recognizes that everything begins with that single customer—whether physician, patient, employer, or insurer—and it involves that customer in every design process it undertakes.

The Importance of Good Partnering

Agile health care systems continually form and re-form partnerships as they respond to changes in the marketplace. In every opportunity to partner, the question to be answered is, How will partnering with *this* organization at *this* time in *this* way create new mutual benefits? What criteria should potential partners apply to themselves and to others identifying that a proposed partnership will work to their mutual advantage? A satisfactory set of criteria will expose the often unspoken but fundamental commitments, expectations, and values that participants in a joint effort typically bring with them.

One approach to selecting potential partners is to assess the core competencies of all of the candidate organizations. An organization must ask itself, "What do we do best? What do we need to continue to own as a core competency in order to remain competitive, and what core competencies do we simply need access to, without the cost of building and maintaining them? Which competencies could we outsource, and which could we cost-effectively partner to obtain?"

Selecting the right partners to participate in an agile collaboration is key to the future success of the enterprise. Once the strategic objectives for the collaboration have been defined, each proposed partner should be selected for the distinctive competency that it can supply to achieve those objectives. When Magee Women's Hospital in Pittsburgh made a strategic decision to extend its continuum of care for high-risk neonates, it looked for partners with core competencies in a variety of fields, such as early childhood education, social assessment, and family counseling, to collaborate in the development of the extended enterprise.

Many hospitals have learned, to their regret, that simply buying up physicians' practices in an effort to capture referrals does not automatically lead to greater income or to competitive advantage in their markets. On the contrary, this strategy has proved ill advised in many cases and for many reasons, not the least of which is that hospitals generally lack a core competency in managing private practices.

Viewing the doctor-hospital relationship from the perspective of the mutual advantage of all stakeholders changes the nature of the relationship. Michael Barton's description in Chapter Three of the PriCare model shows one outcome of such a changed perspective, but others are equally valid, depending on the organizations involved. Lake Hospital, in Painesville, Ohio, has created a fifty-fifty partnership with a group of physicians in which the physicians continue to own and operate their practices but with their success more closely coupled to Lake's. In this instance, the hospital administration acknowledged that the physicians knew more about the management of their practices than they did and that the benefits of this collaboration would be maximized if each partner continued to do what it did best, with the common objective of joint success.

Agile health care organizations, and the collaboration they entail, will evolve to the extent that the collaborating organizations are willing and able to share information, resources, and business process design. It is likely that each party will come to the table with its own discrete set of processes and that, for reasons of cost and comfort, each will try to protect these processes. But agile collaborations depend on enterprise-wide sharing of common processes to facilitate rapid response to customer demands. Thus, as integrated health care alliances are designed, it will be necessary to determine which processes best serve the network as a whole, which need to be adapted, and which need to be discarded in favor of more effective means.

The Virtual Organization Model

Competing on the basis of offering customers dynamic solutions rather than static products requires more than flexible production, operational efficiency, and rapid response. What is needed is an organizational model keyed to the distinctive requirements of creating, producing, and marketing solutions. One of these requirements, reflecting the roles that speed and knowledge play in solutions, is working interactively with employees, customers, suppliers, partners, and even competitors in order to stimulate innovative synergies that benefit everyone by creating wealth that all can share. That is the rationale underlying the emergence of the interprise.

Rather than continuing to function only as stand-alone entities, however integrated with other stand-alone entities, companies are pursuing the ability to use existing resources—from design through field service to the recycling of discarded products and the recovery of production assets—regardless of where the resources are located or who owns them. This would allow each company involved to leverage only those world-class human and technological resources it already possesses that are appropriate to offering customers new solutions.

In effect, companies that are evolving into interprises already have created all of the elements of a virtual organization capability: as a by-product of adapting to new market forces by becoming agile. The virtual organization rises on foundations laid by the market-driven need for agility. It emerges not as someone's great idea of what companies *ought* to do but as a synthesis of the capabilities that companies acquired in response to the value that markets place on speed and solutions.

The virtual organization is an opportunistic, selective integration of distributed human and physical resources into a functional business capability. The distribution can be within a company or among a group of collaborating companies so that virtual organizations can be internal or external. The "product" of the virtual organization can be a single function, such as outpatient surgery, health education, or lab services, or a complete solution, requiring the integration of people possessing all of the competencies required to create, produce, and support the initial solution and its evolution over time.

Virtual organizations are more than partnerships or joint ventures. Their novelty lies in achieving integration by bytes rather than by bricks. This has a number of consequences that are very different from traditional forms of collaboration.

With increasingly sophisticated communication and information technologies, competencies can remain physically distributed even as they are functionally integrated electronically. People with expertise in design, development, production, marketing, sales, service, logistics, finance, facilities management, or human resources can be linked into coordinated working teams whose composition changes as the product or solution they are working on evolves.

For an agile enterprise, the cost of virtual integration is far lower, and the time it takes to create it is far shorter, than physical integration. The human and physical resources commitment required of each participant is sharply limited. Participation in one or more virtual organizations is quite consistent with an organization's, or a department within a company, concurrently going about its daily business. Because the costs are low and the commitment limited, virtual organizations are relatively painless to dissolve if the market opportunity or the project fails to meet expectations.

Solutions typically follow a rapidly evolving marketplace trajectory. The competencies required to continue adding new value for customers also change rapidly, and often unpredictably, driven by new application ideas and new technologies. With a virtual organization, people and organizations with required competencies can be added to or dropped from membership in a timely, efficient, and cost-effective way.

The virtual organization model allows companies with complementary resources and expertise to reduce the sunk costs and risk involvement in new product development, while simultaneously reducing development time. It can help a company with an idea for a new product gain access to customers and distribution channels in markets that it does not serve and in which it has no experience. In addition to reducing time to market, the virtual organization also encourages new product development, a desirable characteristic in a marketplace that is changing rapidly and unpredictably, but expensive if a company guesses wrong about what customers *will* want. And the experience of virtual integration—again, whether internal or external—creates interdependencies, mutual understanding, and transfer of knowledge, all of which encourage further collaboration in other projects.

The virtual organization is a means, not an end. Before adopting it, a company with a new solution concept to transform into a cash stream needs to be confident that it has the supporting infrastructure required. It also needs to be able to make a business case for not developing the new solution all by itself or through a traditional partnership arrangement.

Whether internal or external, virtual organizations require above all else an information, communication, and evaluation environment that values collaboration. The technology requirements are modest by comparison with the managerial environment and the culture of values that it promotes. The drive to use the virtual organization model and overcome the obstacles that are endemic to all traditional enterprises must come from the marketplace.

The Visa credit card is a prototype virtual organization. There is no Visa corporation, nor is there a building or staff commensurate with the size of the operation. Visa is a name for a consortium of over two thousand banks that agree to observe a set of common information and back-office processing protocols. This allows them to treat Visa card carriers as if they were customers of all of the branches of all of those banks. There is a small building and a small staff whose job is coordination of the services that the banks choose to offer and the distributed execution of the tasks necessary to support those services (for example, transaction processing).

There are many reasons that forming virtual organizations may provide significant advantages in the health care industry. For instance, one or more providers may selectively partner to share infrastructure resources, research and development functions, and other costs while simultaneously spreading risk among the partners. Such partnerships provide linkages of complementary core competencies that enable each partner to access all such competencies while eliminating the need for every partner to develop and own the same core competencies.

In Philadelphia, Jefferson Hospital, Pennsylvania Hospital, and the Wills Eye Hospital created a successful virtual neurosurgical service, the largest on the East Coast. Wills had excess room capacity (because of the migration of much of eye surgery to an outpatient service) and underused resources. Jefferson and Pennsylvania hospitals had rival clinical neurosurgical departments with many duplicated facilities. By virtually integrating the full spectrum of professional competencies and support services, patients receive even higher-quality care at lower cost to the provider organizations. The high costs of residency programs for training the next generation of neurosurgeons and constantly developing new surgical and diagnostic capabilities are spread over a much larger base. What had been rivalry has become collaboration. Furthermore, the integration proved robust enough to survive the merger of Pennsylvania Hospital into the University of Pennsylvania Hospital system; it is now a Jefferson-Wills virtual service and still the largest such service on the East Coast.

Another advantage of the virtual organization is its potential to reduce concept-to-cash time. To develop and launch a comprehensive infant and early childhood intervention and education center for a three-county region would require many months and significant investment of personnel and fiscal resources if undertaken by a single hospital. But if several hospitals, neonatal intensive care units, labs, magnetic resonance imaging facilities, social services agencies, day care centers, and public schools were to form a virtual organization—sharing a common strategic plan and a willingness to link their respective business processes—such a center could be developed much more quickly and cost-effectively.

The ability to create a virtual organization does not justify creating one. Obvious questions need to be answered first in order to build a compelling business case for using a virtual production organization rather than one's own. The following is a first-order checklist of questions to which answers must be in hand before an informed decision about the value of the virtual organization model can be reached:

- What is there about the proposed new solution that makes producing it in-house problematic?
- What are the advantages in time and cost in forming a production alliance with other companies?
- What are the relative probabilities of success—meeting the quality, cost, and time-to-market targets—in each approach?
- How high is the price of guessing wrong?
- If an alliance strategy is chosen, who should the allies be?
- How will the anticipated profit be shared, based on the portion of the market value that each partner will add?
- What new expenses will there be in working collaboratively and what new vulnerabilities, for example, to loss of intellectual property?
- What new knowledge might collaboration transfer to the partners' organization, and what proprietary knowledge might each have to share?
- How will the alliance evolve in the face of inevitable changes in customer values?
- How much integration should there be, with whom, and how soon?
- Should an alliance share people, technology, or both, and in what proportion?
- How will the partners establish accountability, and evaluate and reward the performance of the personnel

assigned to a virtual organization project, especially if it is judged to be unsuccessful through no fault of theirs?

- What will take the place of the very important role usually played by a project champion in a single-company product development initiative?
- What metrics will be developed to monitor the success of a virtual organization effort?
- How will quality be monitored?
- Who will deal with residual liability issues after the project is terminated or an organization withdraws?
- How will the partners protect themselves from abuse of intellectual property that must be shared in the joint effort?

The Bottom Line

Here is one difficult truth that every business, including the business of health care, must face in today's economy: *there are no more plateaus*. Change is relentless, and business's response to it must be continuously adaptive.

Clearly many issues still need to be resolved, but the direction for next-generation health care has been set. It will require a flexible, responsive, interactive system that couples the creativity and knowledge of all stakeholders in designing, producing, and delivering total health care solutions to an ever-changing array of health care system opportunities. In short, next-generation health care requires the creation of agile health care organizations. The challenges are great, but the potential rewards are greater. And the future of health care—as a growth business and as a humanitarian service—demands that health care professionals start to think differently about how business is done and service is rendered.

A Systematic Approach to Developing an Agile Organization

This section describes an organization assessment process and a series of exercises that any organization can use to develop and tailor an individualized agility-based action plan. The exercises can be used by a management team—at the department, division, or corporate level—as part of its strategic planning process, by a governing board in a retreat setting, or by representatives of a group of organizations wishing to forge an agile collaboration. We have found that it is helpful if those who wish to employ these exercises have participated in an introductory workshop in agility so that they may begin to work together with a common understanding of agile concepts and principles.

The Agility Forum has created a systematic approach to the development of an agile health care organization using assessment tools and management exercises. The organization seeking to reinvent itself usually needs to get back to basics by first deciding what business it is in or wants to be in. This task often proves much more difficult than it first appears.

Organizational mission statements, for example, typically are of little value, being so broadly written as to be meaningless from a strategic standpoint. Nevertheless, some good examples do exist. When Crozer-Keystone Health System, third largest in the Philadelphia market, decided to rethink its mission, it came up with this: "To manage the health status of the population" of its region. This mission explicitly focuses on health rather than on the treatment of episodic illness. Implicitly, it focuses on long-term relationships with customers to manage their health. It says that the organization will be in partnership with the community it serves to be a resource for all of that community's health-related needs.

Having a clearly articulated vision for the enterprise that is comprehensively shared by all stakeholders, internal and external, is critical to its success. It keeps all the partners focused on a common set of objectives and provides guidance for future decision making.

The series of exercises that follow are based on the facilitated workshop approach developed by the Agility Forum and applied with considerable success to dozens of for-profit and not-for-profit organizations. Typically, these workshops are two days long. Their objective is to formulate a near-term action plan by selectively applying the Forum's generic model of an agile enterprise to the client organization's most pressing problems or most challenging opportunities. Each workshop is thus customized to meet the individual needs of each client, but the process underlying all workshops is the same.

A workshop begins with an exercise that stimulates out-of-the-box thinking about the organization's future success and generates a consensus ranking of the most urgent drivers of change for that organization. The participants are then asked to select, from the forty-two attributes of an agile enterprise in the Forum's four-dimensional model of agility—solutions producer, collaborative operations, adaptive organization, knowledge-driven enterprise—those three attributes whose acquisition would be of the greatest value to their organization. Each of these then becomes the basis for an exercise that creates an implementable action plan leading to the acquisition of that attribute. At the final session of the workshop, the three action plans are critiqued by the group, and decisions are made about responsibilities and a schedule for implementation.

The first exercise is a structured brainstorming session that can be as short as ninety minutes or as long as half a day. It is not necessary to begin the process with this session, but it is an excellent opportunity to prepare the participants for the ideas underlying the exercises that follow.

The next five exercises require that participants prioritize the drivers of change that they perceive their organization to be experiencing and then determine the value to the organization of the attributes of an agile enterprise. (For purposes of these exercises we have condensed the forum's forty-two-attribute model to twenty.) After a brief description by the facilitator of the process and the terminology used, participants can prioritize these twenty attributes on their own time. The group can then meet to collate their individual results and reach a consensus ranking over a working lunch.

In place of the expert facilitators that the forum uses, we have invented a new tool for integrating the results of the prioritization of attributes exercises. The agility compass (see Exercise 7) plots the rankings of the value of the agile enterprise attributes on a traditional compass rose. The result is a visualization of the directions in which an organization, by its own assessment, ought to be pursuing change.

The final exercise is again designed for a structured brainstorming session. Comparing the identification of the most urgent drivers of organizational change and the most important agile attributes to acquire is a reality check. Are the attributes identified as most valuable in fact aligned with the drivers of change judged most urgently in need of a response? They should be and almost always are, but if there *is* a misalignment, that is an important fact about people's perceptions that needs to be confronted. The stage is now set for outlining an action plan for migrating from the status quo to a more agile organization. The final worksheet provides guidance for identifying the steps required by that migration.

Participants in this agility assessment process can be drawn from a single department or, much more valuably, from across departments and functions. Furthermore, once internal personnel have become comfortable with this process, the process could be repeated with external stakeholders. Including representatives of an organization's customer base, as well as key vendors and suppliers, adds considerable value to the results and generates value all by itself.

Regardless of the participant mix, what begins to emerge once the exercises are completed is a consensus view of the organization. The end result is the alignment of individual perceptions with organizational goals and values, as well as the foundation for an agility-based plan of action specific to the organization.

Exercise 1: Six Questions for Agile Organizations

This orientation exercise helps organizations to arrive at a consensus on what will be their reason to exist and their primary market focus. It is best done in a cross-functional group setting where a variety of perspectives and inputs can be elicited. It is in the very diversity of individuals' responses to a common set of questions that the most creative approaches are likely to emerge. An opening exercise that is particularly valuable to people who are rethinking their organization's strategic direction is a focused brainstorming session guided by the six questions that follow. These questions challenge the status quo. They require an organization to begin by examining its customers, for in a truly agile enterprise, all decisions and actions derive from knowing the customers and their needs and expectations. Once these have been clearly identified, a direction for the organization's strategic objectives emerges. An unrelenting discipline focused on building enduring relationships with its customers drives the agile organization.

The commentary following these questions will help to guide the discussion:

1. What business are we really in?
2. Who are our customers? (And our customers' customers?)
3. What do they want? (Do we really know? Do *they* really know?)
4. What is our competition doing better than we are?
5. Are we selling services or solutions? (And which are we *marketing*?)
6. How do we organize differently to identify new customer opportunities, delight existing customers, and optimize resource utilization?

Question 1: What business are we really in? The answer to this first question may seem both obvious and simple, but a group that seriously probes this issue will soon discover how complex it actually is.

The way in which the group members define the business—how they look at it internally, what image they want it to project externally—drives all subsequent decisions. For example, a California health maintenance organization (HMO) found itself struggling to find ways to maximize one of its most profitable products, Medicare gap insurance. Given the federal reimbursement scenario, the HMO recognized that it could not develop any other insurance product to market to seniors. But then someone suggested that they stop thinking of themselves as "an insurance business" and start thinking of themselves as "a senior services business"—and suddenly the possibilities for new products the company could offer to senior citizens was almost unlimited. They began to develop products such as travel insurance and assistance, which allowed them to capitalize on a market they already knew by extending their relationships with their senior customers.

Question 2: Who are our customers? This second question is a natural outgrowth of the first, for once the group decides what business it is in (or wants to be in), it must decide who will need and want its services. How the organization identifies customers will influence what products it develops and how it markets them. Taking that concept one step further, it is important for the group members to understand who their customers' customer is. For example, it has become quite common for hospitals and health care systems to expend enormous marketing budgets on name-recognition advertising. Doubtless this kind of mass media advertising can be effective with informed health care consumers. However, an organization has missed the mark if it is focusing on attracting the patient without also having mounted an effective physician relations effort. The primary customer is now, as ever, physicians—and the patient is *their* customer. It does not matter at all how impressed the patient is with a facility; he or she is not able to self-admit to any hospital or to order an outpatient procedure without a doctor's order. Thus, it is essential for the group to understand who *all* its customers are, and how they relate to the organization and to each other.

Question 3: What do they want? Knowing *who* the customers are is important, but that provides only half of the equation. The group also needs to know what each customer values. Obtaining this information requires direct two-way communication with the customer, using any number of readily available market research tools or by simply engaging the customer in conversation. Many providers still rely primarily on patient satisfaction surveys to gauge their performance. In fact, what many of these surveys measure is not patient satisfaction so much as patient *dis*satisfaction, resulting in a hospital's garnering very little, if any, information about customer-perceived strengths of the organization that could hold potential for creating new business. In this exercise, it is important for the group to explore what it knows about its customers' needs and expectations, and how it knows this information. In today's highly competitive arena, it is not sufficient to have a sense of these things. Rather, reliable data must regularly be gathered, interpreted, and disseminated to those in the organization who can use them to improve services and create products.

Question 4: What is our competition doing better than we are? Seeing the competition with total (even brutal) clarity is essential to defining a market focus. Often it is difficult to be objective about this subject, and many organizations tend to see themselves either as unconquerable superstars in health care or as woefully inadequate underdogs. In fact, neither is likely to be true. What *is* true is that health care players of all stripes need to define their niches if they are to be able to position themselves effectively in the marketplace. Suppose the group knows from reliable market research findings that the competition is gaining market share among referring physicians. It is better to acknowledge the competition's edge and figure out how to respond; ignoring this information is dangerous. Is the competition succeeding because it has electronically linked physician offices to its own lab and medical records departments, thereby facilitating information transmission and retrieval between and among providers? If so, does the group think that its organization can offer similar services? And if it decides not to respond in kind, what other options might it be able to offer physicians that would tie them more closely to the organization? It is also important for the group to know in which areas it may choose *not* to compete. One hospital, located in the shadow of a giant open-heart surgery center, decided to forgo trying to compete in this potentially profitable arena and to concentrate instead on developing the region's largest network of primary care physicians.

Question 5: Are we selling services or solutions? This question looks at services versus solutions and sales versus marketing. A superficial examination of these matters could result merely in a discussion of semantics; in fact, it cuts right to the fundamentals of what the organization's purpose is and how that gets communicated. Too many providers are engaged in producing and delivering episodic care—a single sales transaction that may or may not end with the customer's current need. Hospitals are reimbursed on patient hospital-days, and physicians are paid for performing procedures; hence that is what these providers "sell." Nevertheless, it has become fashionable for providers to characterize themselves as the definitive source for total health care solutions, despite the fact that what they are engaged in is usually a series of single, often random transactions with their customers. Companies may market themselves as solutions providers when in fact they are organized to deliver individual procedures, such as a CT scan, an appendectomy, or a breast cancer screening. These "sales" do not, in fact, provide total solutions but only single services designed to meet an immediate need.

Question 6: How do we organize differently to identify new customer opportunities, delight existing customers, and optimize resource utilization? Frequently there is a serious gap between what an enterprise markets and what it actually sells. The answer to bridging this gap lies in how the enterprise is organized. Today's consumers are demanding total solutions to their problems, from telecommunications to financial services to health care. This trend does not necessarily require that a single organization be capable of managing all the needs of all its customers. It does mean that the enterprise must clearly define which solutions it will provide to which customers, and then adopt the appropriate organizational structure to pursue the strategic initiatives that will enable it to align what it markets with what it sells.

In Chapter Two, Raber and Howgill described one cancer center's effort to provide total cancer care solutions to any patient, with any type of cancer. Solutions entail more than just diagnosis and treatment. As critical as those components are, they alone do not comprise a complete solution. A cancer center organized to provide solutions must provide access to an array of additional services, such as prosthetics, cosmetic resources, psychological and emotional support groups, nutrition counseling, prevention education, and other services that together constitute a total solution to cancer patients' problems. Similarly, a national model for the care of high-risk infants incorporates services not only for neonates but provides a continuum of care that follows these patients into early childhood with education, early intervention programs, and training for parents in all aspects of caring for the special needs of their babies.

The objective of this exercise is to begin the process of opening people's minds to creative thinking about health care organizations. The option of answers that sustain the status quo must be closed off, so that participants are forced to respond by fundamentally rethinking the place of their organization in the health care system—what their organization does versus what it might do, how it operates now versus how it might operate. These open-ended speculations are made more valuable for people in an organization by linking their responses to a series of concrete quantitative assessment exercises that can become the basis for a migration plan to agility.

Exercise 2: Drivers of Change

This exercise requires that each participant identify the specific market forces that are driving change in the organization and prioritize their importance for the organization. Abstracting from national commercial and health care trends, we have organized twenty drivers of organizational change into four broad categories:

Intensifying Competition

Rapidly changing markets

Rapidly changing technologies

Rising pressure on costs and productivity

New competitors

Fragmenting Markets

Need to target niche markets

Low niche market entry costs

Shrinking product lifetimes

Shrinking profit windows

Collaborative Relationships

Inter-enterprise cooperation

Intra-enterprise cooperation

Mergers and consolidation

Outsourcing

Evolving Customer Expectations

Individualized solutions

Changing outcome expectations

Value of information

Social values pressures

Intensifying competition is a battle cry being heard around the world. Markets are changing rapidly, and the pressure on costs and profitability is increasing. At the same time, as Carlson and Hendrickson describe in Chapter Seven, access to information and the latest technologies is becoming ubiquitous. And as Cramer and Lyons underscore in Chapter Six, health care has better-informed consumers than ever before, and they are becoming more demanding all the time. Managed care has created tremendous downward pressures on payments, yet the traditional payment-for-procedures scenario continues to drive costs higher. Advances in technology, such as those being made in telemedicine, put geographically distant competitors next door to one another, thereby eradicating the last barrier to making health care a global commodity.

Fragmentation of mass markets has become the norm in other industries, and it is becoming increasingly common in health care. This reflects the growth of niche markets, the declining cost of entry into those markets, rapidly changing treatment modalities, and shrinking profit margins. As recently as ten years ago the barriers to entry into the magnetic resonance imaging (MRI) market were considerable. Today there seems to be a free-standing MRI center in nearly every neighborhood. Many services formerly delivered only in an acute setting, for example, surgery, rehabilitation, and radiology, are now routinely performed on an outpatient basis in settings far removed from hospitals.

Collaborative business operations is a more recent development in health care, but as a market force it is having enormous impact. Increased outsourcing and resource constraints, interactive vendor-supplier relationships, interactive labor-management relationships, and an emerging trend toward inter-enterprise cooperative agreements are driving consolidation on all fronts. Certainly the trend to outsourcing is well entrenched in hospitals, and core competencies that once would never have been given to outside contractors—such as nursing personnel, accounting and billing functions, and medical department management—are today routinely provided by vendors.

Evolving customer expectations may be one of the most powerful forces driving change in the health care industry. Today's well-informed consumers demand rapid delivery of services, womb-to-

tomb support, and ever-higher levels of care at no additional cost. They have increasingly lofty expectations about health care outcomes ("quality of life" has replaced "survival" as the primary metric of success) and insist on having more input into how, when, and where care is rendered. The rise of consumer activism that has characterized other public arenas—the environment, highway safety, and education, to name a few—now is making itself felt on health care.

The public debate over controversies such as tobacco industry reparations and assisted suicide are only the most extreme examples of the marshaling of public opinion today. HMOs and commercial insurance carriers come under fire daily by consumers unhappy with access, affordability, and coverage, and physicians in private practice are increasingly threatened with malpractice suits brought about by "unsatisfied customers." An agile health care system will recognize all these consumer expectations and will involve customers in the design of its products, services, and delivery modalities. Increasing societal pressures also play into the creation of the agile integrated system. Society continues to make sweeping assumptions about access to and cost of health care. The regulatory environment, always a key factor in health care, becomes ever more rigorous in matters such as waste disposal, cost reimbursement, and consolidation oversight. A thorough understanding of these internal and external pressures will enable the design of a system that is responsive to all its stakeholders.

Worksheet 9.1 measures the relative importance of these market drivers to an organization. Completing this exercise with representatives from as many partnering organizations as possible yields the fullest picture of the challenges the newly created system will face. Analyzing each of these drivers (and adding others that may be in play in specific markets) in terms of the extent to which they affect an organization's goals is the first step toward understanding the external factors influencing an enterprise. Weighting each driver on a scale of 1–5 (with 1 the least important) yields an indication of the degree to which it affects the enterprise. Multiplying the two factors assigns a score of relative importance for each driver.

Worksheet 9.1. Marketplace Drivers

Drivers	Importance to Your Market	Threat to Your Organization	Value to Your Organization
Intensifying Competition			
Rapidly changing markets			
Rapidly changing technologies			
Rising pressure on costs and productivity			
New competitors			
Fragmenting Markets			
Need to target niche markets			
Low niche market entry costs			
Shrinking product lifetimes			
Shrinking profit windows			
Cooperative Relationships			
Inter-enterprise cooperation			
Intra-enterprise cooperation			
Mergers and consolidations			
Outsourcing			
Evolving Customer Expectations			
Individualized solutions			
Changing outcome expectations			
Value of information			
Social values pressures			

Directions: Assign a value from 1 (low) to 5 (high) to the importance of each driver in your market; then assign a value to the threat each driver poses to your organization. Multiply the two numbers together to arrive at a value score for your organization.

Exercise 3: Solutions Producer

In Chapter One, Goldman explains the agility attributes that define an agile organization: solutions producer, collaborative operations, adaptive organization, and knowledge-driven enterprise. This exercise and the following three address these attributes.

Each organization that becomes a partner in an agile system must always be striving to attain these attributes. But for the system as an extended enterprise, even more is required. Once again, the place to start is with the customers, and these customers should be treated as *stakeholders* in the system who have both input and responsibility for its success.

Collaborative health care alliances have many customers, each with their own set of expectations and priorities. Often these expectations and values will be in direct conflict with those of other customers. The patient's expectation, for example, is that health care providers will manage a system of womb-to-tomb coverage. Employers' expectations, on the other hand, are that they will be required to pay as little as possible for this coverage. The insurer's expectation is that providers will render only the most essential care and that they will accept the lowest possible fees for doing so.

If an extended enterprise collaboration is to be successful, it must begin by bringing all of the stakeholders to the table for a full and candid discussion of the explicit and implicit issues relevant to the collaboration. Framing the discussion around how the enterprise will work to achieve the agility attributes described in Chapter One is an effective tactic for keeping participants focused on the "to be" state instead of becoming mired in the political issues of the "as is" state.

Worksheets 9.2 through 9.5 assess the extent to which the organization possesses the highest-level attributes of agility and the value of those attributes for it. Completing these worksheets will result in a prioritized ranking of the agile attributes that participants believe their organization will most benefit from acquiring. Each worksheet has five attributes associated with one of the four dimensions of agility, as described above. For each, the participants assign a value of 1 to 5 (with 1 the lowest value). In the first column of the worksheet, they rank the importance of that attribute to the organization. Would possessing this attribute contribute significantly to its future success (5), be helpful but not critical (3), or is it of marginal importance (1)? In the second column, they rank how well the organization exhibits that attribute at the present time. Is it the routinely well-executed norm (5), a goal occasionally met (3), or a weakness (1)? Finally, in the third column, they enter the product of these two rankings, to obtain a final score for each attribute of between 1 and 25. Once these attributes have been prioritized, they will be plotted on the agility compass in Figure 9.1 to generate a picture of the organization's agile strengths and weaknesses.

As participants fill in Worksheets 9.2 through 9.5, they should keep Worksheet 9.1, with their ranking of the drivers of change at hand. Their evaluation of the relative importance of these drivers establishes a frame of reference for how the organization should prioritize its attributes. When it comes time to generate an action plan, in Exercise 6, the participants can use the drivers worksheet again as a reality check that their proposed plan actually addresses the needs for change identified as most urgent.

The objective of Worksheet 9.2 (and the three that follow) is to assess how far along the road to agility the organization has already journeyed. On each line of these worksheets should be entered a value from 1 to 5 that participants feel best answers the question represented by the line entry:

1.1 *Target niche markets*. To what extent has the organization shifted from targeting mass markets with standardized products and services to targeting niche markets with a wide variety of differentiated products and services?

1.2 *Rapid concept to cash*. How rapidly can the organization bring a compelling idea for a new solution to the marketplace?

Worksheet 9.2. Solutions Producer

	Importance to Your Market ×	Existing Capability =	Value to Your Organization
1.1 Target niche markets			
1.2 Rapid concept to cash			
1.3 Proactive customer relationships			
1.4 Individualized solutions			
1.5 Solutions-based marketing			

Directions: On a scale of 1 to 5 (low to high), rank the importance to your market of each attribute. On the same scale, rank your organization's current capability for each attribute. Finally, multiply the two numbers together to get the value score for your organization.

1.3 *Proactive customer relationships*. To what extent have employees developed proactive relationships with customers in order to understand what they *would* value based on their individual requirements, often in advance of their own realization?

1.4 *Individualized solutions*. If the organization is in fact producing solutions for customers, to what extent have managers changed marketing strategies from a product-service focus to a solution focus? (If this sounds like a "What color was George Washington's white horse?" sort of question, it isn't! Many companies did not coordinate the shift to developing and producing solutions with appropriate shifts in marketing programs and sales force training and compensation until problems arose.)

1.5 *Solutions-based marketing*. To what extent has the organization shifted from selling traditional products and services to offering customers solutions that are tailored to their individual requirements?

Exercise 4: Collaborative Operations

Fill out Worksheet 9.3 in answer to these questions:

2.1 *Cooperation-based operations*. To what extent is cooperation an operational strategy of first choice in the organization? Cooperation can take many forms, of course: internal, among personnel within a single department or division, or across internal organizational boundaries; or external, with suppliers, customers, other potential partners, and other organizations. Underlying all of these is the value placed on cooperation as a preferred way of performing work and creating products and services, rather than a last resort. The question, then, is the extent to which cooperation is valued highly as a routine approach to getting things done.

2.2 *Interactive supplier relationships*. To what extent has the organization developed interactive relationships with suppliers?

2.3 *Electronic commerce interoperability*. To what extent has the organization developed electronic commerce capabilities? At one extreme of this spectrum is simple electronic data interchange; at the other, the ability to engage in the full range of relevant commercial activities electronically: exchanging information with suppliers, customers, and partners via intra- or extranets, with at least core business processes linked electronically to those of selected other organizations. The term *interoperability* refers to the electronic linkages among information systems that allow for the seamless flow of information within and among organizations, independent of the hardware or software being used. (The Internet is an outstanding example of sophisticated interoperability. Users do not have to care about the hardware or software they are using so long as they observe agreed-on protocols, nor do users have to know what hardware and software others are using.)

2.4 *Proactive information sharing*. Cooperation entails sharing information, yet organizations historically have been reluctant to share information except in very controlled ways. To what extent has the organization recognized that sharing information proactively and aggressively with other organizations, such as suppliers, customers, and partners, can promote growth?

2.5 *Virtual organization capability*. The ultimate test of a company's commitment to and capacity for cooperation is its readiness to be part of a virtual organization. To what extent is the organization ready to initiate or accept an invitation to participate in a virtual organization?

Worksheet 9.3. Collaborative Operations

	Importance to Your Market ×	Existing Capability =	Value to Your Organization
2.1 Cooperation-based operations			
2.2 Interactive supplier relations			
2.3 Electronic commerce interoperability			
2.4 Proactive information sharing			
2.5 Virtual organization capability			

Directions: On a scale of 1 to 5 (low to high), rank the importance to your market of each attribute. On the same scale, rank your organization's current capability for each attribute. Finally, multiply the two numbers together to get the value score for your organization.

Exercise 5: Adaptive Organization

Use Worksheet 9.4 to answer the following questions:

3.1 *Motivation-and-support management style*. Command-and-control as a management style made some sense in a rigidly hierarchical organization with centralized authority, in which people did only what they were told to do by their organizational superiors. In an agile organization, command-and-control is simply dysfunctional. To what extent has management in the organization made the shift from command-and-control to motivation-and-support?

3.2 *Decentralized decision making*. A motivation-and-support management style leads to better total organization performance only if it is coupled to a strategy of distributing authority and decentralizing decision making in a coordinated way. The objective in an agile organization is to push decision making down as close to the operational level as possible, consistent with the ability to relate local decisions to their broader organizational impact. To what extent have decision making and authority been decentralized in the organization?

3.3 *Innovative and entrepreneurial workforce*. Decentralized decision making is not worth much if the workforce is passive, waiting to be told what to do and how to do it. Management in an agile organization has two primary responsibilities: motivating the workforce to be entrepreneurial, to "think like an owner" in performing their jobs, and to support the workforce by providing the changing resources they will need to do so. How entrepreneurial, how willing to take the initiative to change what they do and/or how they do it, is the workforce in the organization?

3.4 *Opportunity-driven organization*. A central attribute of an agile organization is that it is able to organize human and physical resources in response to customer opportunities. An agile organization does not have a fixed operational structure, dictated by a rigid organizational hierarchy. Instead, organizational structure is flexible enough to be a means of supporting aggressive responses to marketplace change. To what extent is the organization of work in the organization pulled by market opportunities rather than fixed?

3.5 *Shared risk and reward.* To what extent does the workforce in the organization share in the risks of change and in the rewards of successful change? This is the litmus test of a management-and-support management style. If there is no sharing in the rewards and no accountability for risk taking, empowerment is empty.

Worksheet 9.4. Adaptive Organization

	Importance to Your Market ×	Existing Capability =	Value to Your Organization
3.1 Motivation-and-support management style			
3.2 Decentralized decision making			
3.3 Innovative and entrepreneurial workforce			
3.4 Opportunity-driven organization			
3.5 Shared risk and reward			

Directions: On a scale of 1 to 5 (low to high), rank the importance to your market of each attribute. On the same scale, rank your organization's current capability for each attribute. Finally, multiply the two numbers together to get the value score for your organization.

Exercise 6: Knowledge-Driven Organization

Use Worksheet 9.5 to answer the following questions:

4.1 *Competency-based strategic planning*. In a truly knowledge-driven organization, strategic planning is keyed to the competencies of the workforce, to what they know and know how to do: knowledge they currently possess that can be built on, knowledge that must be added now (for example, by recruiting, partnering, or acquisition), and knowledge that will be needed in the workforce in the near and middle term. To what extent is strategic planning in the organization keyed to knowledge as the organization's core competitive asset?

4.2 *Knowledge management processes*. To what extent has the organization implemented processes for capturing the knowledge of the workforce, acquiring new knowledge, and managing its systematic organization and dissemination to everyone who could create value by using knowledge innovatively?

4.3 *Adaptive information system*. How flexible is the information system in evolving as information and knowledge management requirements evolve?

4.4 *Open information and communication environment*. To what extent is there an open information and communication environment in the organization, reflecting management's commitment to supporting the objective of a knowledgeable, entrepreneurial workforce motivated to create new solutions continually?

4.5 *Continuous and cross-functional education and training*. In a knowledge-driven organization, education and training are an investment in continuing competitiveness. A hallmark of agility is the recognition that education and training—for many organizations, cross-functional education and training—are not a cost but an investment, and that they must be continuous and open to everyone, not just to professionals. To what extent is the organization committed to continuous education and training and, if it is (or would be) relevant, to cross-functional education and training?

Exercise 7: Creating an Action Plan

The data generated by completing these worksheets implicitly define an Agility Compass, pointing to the direction that a particular organization, confronting changing demands and opportunities, needs to take to become agile. As these demands and opportunities change continually, rapidly, and often unpredictably, an agile organization expects continually to reexamine the adaptation of its organizational and operational attributes to its competi-

Worksheet 9.5. Knowledge-Driven Organization

	Importance to Your Market ×	Existing Capability =	Value to Your Organization
4.1 Competency-based strategic planning			
4.2 Knowledge management processes			
4.3 Adaptive information system			
4.4 Open information and communication environment			
4.5 Continuous and cross-functional education and training			

Directions: On a scale of 1 to 5 (low to high), rank the importance to your market of each attribute. On the same scale, rank your organization's current capability for each attribute. Finally, multiply the two numbers together to get the value score for your organization.

tive environment and implement appropriate changes. The only constant, then, is the regular need to revisit exercises such as the ones described here.

The information in Worksheets 9.2 through 9.5 can be visualized by plotting the twenty responses around the four strategic capabilities of an agile organization, as in Figure 9.1. On such a plot, a perfectly agile organization would have the shape of a circle with a radius of 25: the product of a ranking of 5 for the value of the attribute and a ranking of 5 for possessing it fully. Deviations from circularity reveal a deviation from agility. At the same time, they define the goals of an action plan for migrating to agility.

Any sound action plan must answer the following questions:

1. What actions are to be taken?
2. Why?
3. What resources will be required to implement them?
4. How are they to be implemented?
5. What obstacles can be anticipated?
6. How are the obstacles to be overcome?
7. What is the time frame for implementation?

The responses to Worksheets 9.2 through 9.5 are the basis for answering the first question. The responses to Worksheet 9.1 provide a basis for answering the second question. Participants should review the values that they assigned to the sixteen generic drivers of organizational change in Worksheet 9.1, select the three highest-ranking drivers of change for their organization, and enter them in the first part of Worksheet 9.6.

Participants then review the values that they assigned to the twenty attributes listed in Worksheets 9.2 through 9.6 and select the three attributes that their organization would most benefit from acquiring or becoming more proficient at. In general, these will be the three attributes with the highest importance value and the lowest

Figure 9.1. The Agility Compass

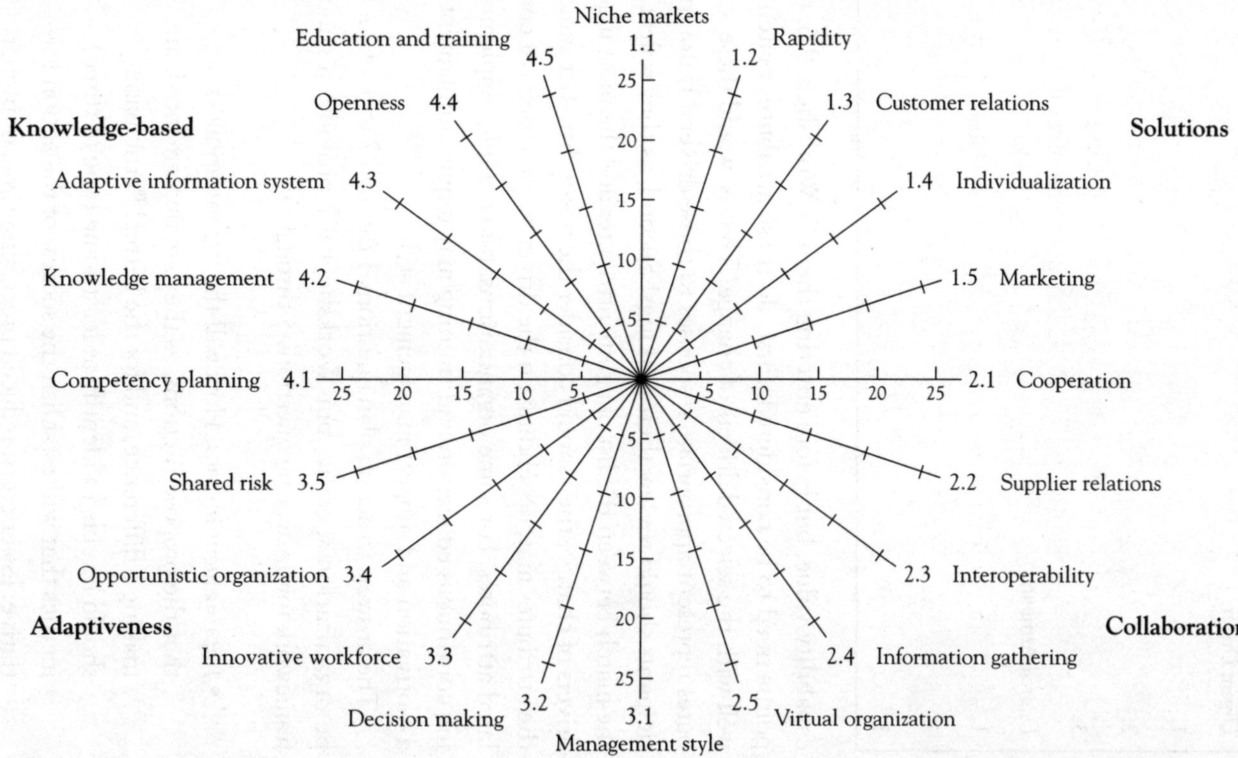

Worksheet 9.6. Alignment of Drivers and Attributes

Urgent Drivers
1.
2.
3.
Desired Attributes
1.
2.
3.

capability value, but before entering them in Worksheet 9.6, two points need to be considered. First, do these attributes match up well with the selected drivers of change? That is, would these attributes represent appropriate responses to those drivers? If not, participants should review their rankings! Second, as they reflect on the match between the list of agility attributes and the most urgent drivers of change, they should consider the possibility that some of the attributes may, depending on the driver, form clusters of correlated attributes. For some organizations, for example, implementing continuous education and training may require implementing a motivation and support management style.

The answers to action plan questions 3 through 7 will, of course, be organization specific, but Worksheet 9.7 provides a general framework for answering questions 3 through 5:

- *Improvement metrics*. How will the organization know that the proposed actions, as they are implemented, are making a difference, and for the better? Participants should be able to identify at least some (one to three) metrics that will establish the success of the action initiative: lower costs, reduced processing time, or higher market share, for example.

Worksheet 9.7. Building an Action Plan

Improvement metrics

1.

2.

3.

Business process changes

1.

2.

3.

Organizational structure changes

1.

2.

3.

Human resource changes

1.

2.

3.

Technology changes

1.

2.

3.

Leadership issues

1.

2.

3.

- *Business process changes*. What changes in current business processes will be required if this action plan is to be implemented?
- *Organizational structure changes*. What changes in the current organizational structure will be required?
- *Human resource changes*. What human resource changes will be required?
- *Technology changes*. What technology changes will be required?
- *Leadership issues*. What leadership issues will need to be addressed?

The Rewards of Making the Effort

Becoming agile is neither as difficult nor as obvious as it may at first appear. Without unqualified management commitment and a well-thought-out strategic plan, a company will not become agile naturally. Organizations will fail for lack of making the effort, or will find the transition painful and costly in human as well as in financial terms if the effort is uncoordinated, poorly conceived, or half-hearted. On the other hand, with strong support from management, proper planning, and a correct understanding of the logic of the current commercial environment, any organization can become *more* agile. And to the extent that it is open to learning from the experiences of other organizations, the transition will be less painful and less costly.

References

American Management Association and Tierney & Partners. "Business Use of the Internet: An Executive Assessment." Executive summary. New York: AMA, 1997.

Ashkenas, B., Ulrich, D., Jick, T., and Kerr, S. *The Boundaryless Organization: Breaking the Chains of Organizational Structure*. San Francisco: Jossey-Bass, 1995.

Bischof, R. O., Smith, R. L., Nash, D. B., Murray, J. F., Louis, D. Z., Hanchak, N. A., and Schlackman, N. "Bridging the Gap Between Managed Care and Academic Medicine: An Innovative Fellowship." *American Journal of Managed Care*, 1997, *3*(1), 107–111.

Blumenthal, D., and Thier, S. O. "Managed Care and Medical Education: The New Fundamentals." *Journal of the American Medical Association*, Sept. 4, 1996, pp. 725–727.

Cohen, J. J. "Learning to Care, for a Healthier Tomorrow." *Academic Medicine*, 1996, *71*(2), 121–125.

Cohen, J. J., and Whitcomb, M. E. "Are the Recommendations of the AAMC's Task Force on the Generalist Physician Still Valid?" *Academic Medicine*, 1997, *72*(1), 13–16.

Collins, J. C., and Porras, J. I. *Built to Last: Successful Habits of Visionary Companies*. New York: HarperCollins, 1994.

Collins, J. C., and Porras, J. I. "Building Your Company's Vision." *Harvard Business Review*, Sept.–Oct. 1996, p. 65.

D'Alessandro, M., and others. "The Virtual Hospital: An IAIMS Integrating Continuing Education into the Work Flow." *MD Computing*, 1996, *13*(4), 323–329.

DePalma, D. A., McCarthy, J. C., Raffetto, B. A., and MacKenzie, M. L. "Web Best Practices." Interactive Technology Strategies series, vol. 2, no. 4. Cambridge, Mass.: Forrester Research Group, 1997.

Eisenberg, D. M., Kessler, R. C., Foster, C., Norlock, F. E., Calkins, D. R., and Delbanco, T. L. "Unconventional Medicine in the United States: Prevalence, Costs, and Patterns of Use." *New England Journal of Medicine*, Jan. 28, 1993, pp. 246–252.

Elliott, J. "Managed Care Spices Up: The 1996 HIMSS/HP Leadership Survey." *Health Care Informatics*, 1996, *13*(5), special supplement, p. 4.

Elliott, R. L., Juthani, N. V., Rubin, E. H., Greenfield, D., Skelton, W. D., and Yudkowsky, R. "Quality in Residency Training: Toward a Broader, Multidimensional Definition." *Academic Medicine*, 1996, *71*(3), 243–248.

Erikson, E. *Youth and Crisis*. New York: Norton, 1968.

"Experts Explore Emerging Technologies' Effects on Medicine." *Journal of the American Medical Association*, Mar. 6, 1996.

Friedman, J. H. *An Overview of Predictive Learning and Functional Approximation*. Technical Report no. 112. Stanford, Calif.: Stanford University, 1994.

Gage, J. S. "An Introduction to JAVA." *MD Computing*, 1996, *13*(6), 476.

Goldberg, D. E. *Genetic Algorithms in Search, Optimization and Machine Learning*. Reading, Mass.: Addison-Wesley, 1986.

Herzlinger, R. *Market Driven Health Care: Who Wins, Who Loses in the Transformation of America's Largest Service Industry*. Reading, Mass.: Addison-Wesley, 1997.

Jefferson Medical College. *Annual Report 1995–1996*. Philadelphia: Thomas Jefferson University.

Jefferson Medical College. Sophomore Seminar Series: Contemporary Issues in Medicine, 1997–1998.

Kobayashi, T., and others. "Effect of a Computer-Aided Diagnosis Scheme on Radiologists' Performance in Detection of Lung Nodules on Radiographs." *Radiology*, 1996, *199*, 843–848.

Kotter, J. P. "What Leaders Really Do." *Harvard Business Review*, May–June 1990.

Lopez, M. "Data Repository: Vision Becomes Reality." *Health Care Informatics*, 1996, *13*(1), 61–62.

Louis, D. Z., and Nash, D. B. *Health Policy: An Introduction to the Health Care System*. Philadelphia: Jefferson Medical College, 1997.

Lurie, N. "Preparing Physicians for Practice in Managed Care Environments." *Academic Medicine*, 1996, *71*(10), 1044–1049.

Maccoby, M. *The Gamesman*. New York: Simon & Schuster, 1976.

March, E. L., and Moore, G. T. "Allied for Good: Academic Medicine and Managed Care Form Educational Partnerships." *New Medicine*, Fall 1997, pp. 179–182.

Morris, B. "He's Nice. He's Not Nice. He's Saving Big Blue." *Fortune*, Apr. 14, 1997, p. 71.

Murray, R. B., and Tawyea, E. *Building a Global Education Network*. Philadelphia: Academic Information Services & Research, Thomas Jefferson University, 1996.

1997 Learning Infrastructure Project Report. Philadelphia: Thomas Jefferson University, 1997.

Olson, R. "Information Technology in Home Health Care." In C. Bezold and E. Mayer (eds.), *Future Care: Responding to the Demand for Change*. New York: Faulkner & Gray, 1996

Ozbolt, J. "From Minimum Data to Maximum Impact: Using Clinical Data to Strengthen Patient Care." *MD Computing*, 1997, *14*(4), 295–300.

Partnerships for Quality Education. *Learning Together*. Philadelphia: Partnerships for Quality Education, 1997.

Partnerships for Quality Education. *Narrative Report to the Pew Charitable Trusts*. Philadelphia: Partnerships for Quality Education, Jun. 1997.

Phillips, R. R., Lee, M. Y., Berman, H. A., and Madoff, M. A. "The Tufts Partnership for Managed Care Education." *Academic Medicine*, May 1997, pp. 347–356.

Preiss, K., Goldman, S., and Nagel, R. N. *Cooperate to Compete: Building Agile Business*. New York: Van Nostrand Reinhold, 1996.

Prokesch, S. E. "Competing on Customer Service: An Interview with British Airway's Sir Colin Marshall." *Harvard Business Review*, Nov.–Dec. 1995, p. 108.

Ramo, J. D. "Doc in a Box." *Time*, 1996, *148*(14), 55.

Renner, K. "Electronic Medical Records in the Outpatient Setting." MGM *Journal*, 1996, *43*(3), 52–74.

Riesman, D. *The Lonely Crowd: A Study of the Changing American Character*. New Haven, Conn.: Yale University Press, 1950.

Roberts, B. "Lots of Data Types, One Front End." *Webweek*, 1996, *2*(12), 27, 30.

Robinson, A. L. "The Buyers Health Care Action Group: Creating a Competitive Care System Model." *Managed Care Quarterly*, 1997, 5, 61.

Schneider, P. "Consult an Expert: Your Computer." *Health Care Informatics*, 1996a, *13*(5), 37, 40.

Schneider, P. "CPR Distinction: Three Organizations Furthering the Cause." *Health Care Informatics*, 1996b, *13*(6) 120–126.

Schneider, P. "The Quest for Intelligence." *Health Care Informatics*, 1996c, *13*(10), 69–70.

Schneider, P. "Computerized Quality Checks Yield Savings." *Health Care Informatics*, 1997, *14*(5), 3.

Shine, K. I. "Educating Physicians for the Real World." In E. Ginsburg (ed.), *Urban Medical Centers: Balancing Academic and Patient Care Functions*. Boulder, Colo: Westview Press, 1996.

Sullivan, M. "The CPR's Hidden Impact: Reducing Malpractice Risk." *Health Care Informatics*, 1996, *13*(6) 36–38.

Tam, T. A. "Allina Health System's Approach to High Tech and High Touch." *Managed Care Quarterly*, 1997, *5*, 59.

Tichy, N., and Charan, R. "Speed, Simplicity and Self-Confidence: An Interview with Jack Welch." *Harvard Business Review*, Sept. 1, 1989.

University of Arizona. Program in Integrative Medicine. Fellowship description in program brochure, 1997.

Veloski, J., Barzansky, B., Nash, D. B., Bastacky, S., and Stevens, D. P. "Medical Student Education in Managed Care Settings: Beyond HMOs." *Journal of the American Medical Association*, Sept. 4, 1996, pp. 667–671.

Wager, K. A., Ornstein, S. M., and Jenkins, R. G. "Perceived Value of Computer-Based Patient Records Among Clinician Users." *MD Computing*, 1997, *14*(5) 334.

Wartman, S. A. "Managed Care and Its Effect on Residency Training in Internal Medicine." *Archives of Internal Medicine*, 1994, *154*, 2539–2544.

Wennberg, J. E., and Cooper, M. M. *The Dartmouth Atlas of Health Care*. Chicago: American Hospital Publishing, 1998.

White, C., and Hemby, C. "Automating the Bedside." *Health Care Informatics*, 1997, *14*(2), 68.

Whyte, W. *The Organization Man*. New York: Simon & Schuster, 1956.

Zaleznik, A. "Managers and Leaders: Are They Different?" *Harvard Business Review*, May–June 1977.

Index